ARKANA

# HUMAN ENERGY SYSTEMS

Jack Schwarz, a pioneer in the education health field, has gained worldwide recognition for his work. He is the president of the Aletheia Foundation, which he founded in 1958, and has been a subject, researcher, and consultant at major bio-medical and life science research centers in the United States and abroad. Results of tests performed on Jack document his abilities to self-regulate many psycho-physiological processes.

Jack Schwarz is dedicated to educating others in self-health and awareness, and bringing together research on health and human energies. *The Power of Personal Health*, also available in Arkana, is the latest in a series of books in which he explores the dynamics of health education, always with an emphasis on energy and self-regulation.

For further information on Jack Schwarz and the Aletheia Foundation, contact: Aletheia Foundation, 515 N.E. 8th Street, Grants Pass, OR 97526; (503) 479-4855.

# HUMAN
# ENERGY
# SYSTEMS

## Jack Schwarz

Published in Association with

Robert Briggs

ARKANA

DEDICATED TO

*Lois A. Scheller for being a true partner*
*and for constantly providing the balance between*
*the Yin and the Yang.*

ARKANA
Published by the Penguin Group
Viking Penguin, a division of Penguin Books USA Inc.,
375 Hudson Street, New York, New York 10014, U.S.A.
Penguin Books Ltd, 27 Wrights Lane,
London W8 5TZ, England
Penguin Books Australia Ltd, Ringwood,
Victoria, Australia
Penguin Books Canada Ltd, 10 Alcorn Avenue, Suite 300,
Toronto, Ontario, Canada M4V 3B2
Penguin Books (N.Z.) Ltd, 182–190 Wairau Road,
Auckland 10, New Zealand

Penguin Books Ltd, Registered Offices:
Harmondsworth, Middlesex, England

First published in the United States of America by E. P. Dutton 1980
Published in Arkana Books 1992

1  3  5  7  9  10  8  6  4  2

THE LIBRARY OF CONGRESS HAS CATALOGUED THE ORIGINAL EDITION AS FOLLOWS:

Schwarz, Jack
Human energy systems.
1. Occult sciences. 2. Aura.
3. Materia medica, Vegetable. I. Title.
BF1999.S362    1979    001.9    79-12835
ISBN: 0-525-48301-2 (Dutton)
ISBN: 0 14 019.355 3 (Penguin)

Printed in the United States of America

# Contents

# Acknowledgments

**THANKS TO**

Dr. Elmer Green and his wife Dr. Alyce Green for their fine Foreword and their continuous support.

Bill Whitehead for being a most understanding and enthusiastic senior editor. Pat Murray for her excellence in finalizing the manuscript. Kathy Goss for unscrambling the material with patient and tedious pre-editing. Robert Briggs for his assistance in getting this book published.

Lois A. Scheller for being there at all times and giving me the chance of accomplishment.

All my students who have shared their insights with me.

# Foreword

In 1972 when Jack Schwarz first visited our Psychophysiology Laboratory at The Menninger Foundation, we did not know what he was capable of doing or what he wished to demonstrate. Paul Herbert, an astute observer, had told me (E. G.) in the early part of the year that in his experience a certain Dutchman by the name of Jack Schwarz was more talented than most of the yogis coming to California. But that was the extent of our knowledge. At Paul's suggestion, I called Jack Schwarz and told him we would be pleased to show him our laboratory if at some future date he happened to be passing through Kansas. Several months later Jack phoned and said he wished to accept my invitation and could arrive at the Kansas City airport on November 30 and stay until December 8. I looked doubtfully at our research schedule, but saw that those days were open—the only free ones for several weeks—so I agreed.

In *Beyond Biofeedback* (Delacorte Press, 1977), we have written about Jack's subsequent demonstrations of pain and bleeding control, his "reading" of auras, his visualization technique for "communicating with the body." We also wrote about the problem of discriminating between "seeing" and "projecting" and made a few comments on the misunderstandings that arise between scientists and mystics, between the analytic and the intuitive modes of perception.

It is on this difficult subject of rational versus intuitive that we wish now to focus—for unless this problem is understood, there is no easy way for people who are primarily rational and analytic, but not intuitive, to understand Jack Schwarz. Understanding is especially difficult for these people because Jack laces his discussions with down-to-earth analogies that, because of the multidimensional nature of our cosmos, can never be exact. His verbal skill is, in a certain way, an obstacle for analytic listeners. His analogies are valuable for those who are *not* analytically minded or burdened with scientific learning, however, because such analogies guide the intuition, often eliciting unexpected flashes of insight.

For the purely analytical thinker (biochemical, Freudian, or whatever), much of what Jack says has a different meaning from what he means. How can this be? The reason is deeply metaphysical, based on the notion that when you put an experience into words, it is already wrong. And Jack is an experientialist, an existentialist, a mystic, an occultist—not a scientist. He is concerned with the "separate reality," as Don Juan would put it, expressed in analogies drawn from our ordinary reality, and this is the problem. We are not revealing anything here of which Jack himself is not fully aware, but unless the reader knows this in advance, prejudgment can interfere with understanding.

It is relevant here to mention the basic difference between science and intuition, between left and right hemispheres of the brain (to use a popular metaphor). As everyone knows, the scientific concept of the way the universe is arranged is actually a model we have constructed in our minds. In terms of brain, we try to describe the cosmos by means of a left cortex model. In *Science and Sanity*, Alfred Korzybski, the father of general semantics, examines this problem of intellectual models in depth. He compares our models of the universe to maps and points out that no matter how faithfully maps follow contours, they are not the terrain. On the other hand, from a right cortex point of view, a nonanalytical, see-it-as-a-whole point of view, the terrain is something to experience, not to make maps of. This difference in mode of perception seems to account for some of the basic conflicts between intellect and intuition, between scientist and mystic, and this difference is not easy to bridge if one's intellectual sophistication is fully developed before any awareness of "a separate reality" develops. After intellectual sophistication has "hardened," it is often difficult to enlarge the frame of reference sufficiently to contemplate the kinds of things Jack Schwarz talks about. On the other hand, if a person has developed from a young age into parapsychological sophistication, so that the "separate reality" has primary significance and ordinary reality appears only as a special case, or cross section of the other, then it is usually difficult for that person to compress his or her logic into ordinary Euclidian and Aristotelian modes.

Most people are unaware of the fact that in science, *certainty* about any subject of discussion is approached only by disproving alternate hypotheses; in statistics this is specifically recognized as "disproving the *null* hypotheses." To prove a book is on the table it is necessary to prove that it is nowhere else—an impossible task. This may seem foolish to the literal minded, but it results from the nature of our ordinary reality and ordinary logic. That is the way it is. After all, the book could be a holographic projection. All the sensory systems of the body can be misled in one way or another. Seeing is not believing.

In the intuitive domain, however, certainty often seems to precede factual knowledge. Perhaps that is why some scientists will not yet accept the possibility that perception of "a separate reality" might exist in anyone. They debate the existence of the perceptions themselves.

Imagine a biology class in which a frog is being studied with a scanner that shows continuously, on a video screen, a single expanded cross section of the creature, including microscopic detail of various organs, with a line of skin as a boundary. (A somewhat similar device is already in use, of course, making brain and body scans in hospitals.) Now, imagine that in this biology class the lights are always off and the only thing that has ever been visible to students is the video screen. The frog is observed only as a single two-dimensional cross section on the video screen, changing continuously in dozens of macroscopic and microscopic details.

What, then, would students learn about a frog? Many consistent relationships between parts would be noted, of course, and a logic and mathematics would eventually be developed to describe these consistencies; but what would students really understand about the nature of frogs in our present world?

Now, imagine that one of the students takes his eyes from the video screen, turns on a flashlight, looks at the frog and realizes that the scanning device and all the associated hardware are part of a "sensory system" that mechanically develops a limited cross-sectional view of the animal. How would this student then describe what he saw to the others? What words would he use to describe his perceptions? Naturally, he would have to use two-dimensional references and analogies to explain the three-dimensional actuality and he would fail with many of his associates. Possibly he would be called a mystic, in either complimentary or disparaging ways depending on what individual students were able to "see." (In this case, it might depend on whether or not the others had flashlights.)

This example illustrates the contradictory situation in which scientists and mystics often find themselves. Scientists describe the cosmos in four-dimensional terms (including time) and mystics describe a universe with additional dimensions and use ordinary four-dimensional words in trying to get their meanings across. Tibetan Buddhists long ago abandoned that approach and began to refer to the universe of other dimensions as the Void, not because those dimensions were void of substance and actuality, but because the perceptual systems developed by most humans perceived nothing there. W. Y. Evans-Wentz's Tibetan teacher, who helped him translate the *Tibetan Book of the Dead,* said there were twenty-eight different kinds of experience in the Void, none of them open to time-and-space awareness.

This problem of differing awareness has been discussed through the ages by mystics, seers, and thinkers in all philosophies and religions. This is Jack Schwarz's problem in trying to describe his universe of perception. Scientists often describe in mathematical terms what they perceive with their physical faculties and with instrumental extensions of those faculties, and in so describing the universe are often wrong, but for the "right" reasons. Those who tend to perceive directly with their mental apparatus, perceiving in beyond-space-time dimensions, are unable by the nature of perception and language to develop a correct verbal structure. Verbal structure, having been created for space-time, is by definition inadequate and misleading. As a result, intuitives are often right, but for the wrong reasons.

Because of the difficulty in thinking about a multidimensional cosmos, readers might usefully follow Korzybski's advice in *Science and Sanity.* Near the beginning of his book the author points out that he uses words in new ways and that there is no way to define the words in advance because the meanings depend on how they are used. Therefore, he says, it is necessary to read the book once to find out what the words mean, and then read it a second time to find out what the text means. This suggestion can well be applied by analytically-minded people when they read the present book. The words Jack uses, selected from our ordinary reality, are not adequate. He describes a reality that seems to have more dimensions than the cosmos with which we are familiar. Unless we find out how he uses the words, it is inevitable that we will not know what he is talking about.

For instance, physicists and engineers will be confused on the first page by the following sentence: "The magnetic aspect of our energy fields has to do with our being in the physical world; for example, it is what keeps us upright." Our advice to the reader of this passage is to hold the idea in memory for future reference without feeling immediately driven to know its meaning. This process is remarkably useful for reading in the existential domain, where words are inadequate, where a new awareness often must be developed before communication can be satisfactory. This approach is also necessary because Jack, not trained as a scientist, uses words in the popular rather than the scientific mode.

Perseverance is necessary; impatience is inappropriate. Remember that it took Don Juan some thirteen years to train his anthropologist student, Carlos Castaneda, and during a large part of that time Castaneda wrestled with the task of integrating the experiential and the intellectual.

Having said that, we wish the reader all the best, and an exciting journey.

ELMER GREEN, ALYCE GREEN

*Topeka, Kansas*

# 1 : Human Energy Fields

**Measuring the Human Energy Output**

With progress in modern science, we are becoming more and more aware that the human organism is not just a physical structure made up of molecules, that we are electrochemical and electromagnetic beings made up of energy fields. Our bodies may appear to be solid and opaque, but if we could magnify the cells, molecules, and atoms of which we are composed, we would see that at the most fundamental level we are made up of energy, of electrochemical and electromagnetic activity that is constantly going on in our bodies.

If electricity is the force behind our electromagnetic energy fields, then magnetism is the direction-giving aspect of that force. The magnetic aspect of our energy fields has to do with our functioning in the physical world; for example, it is what keeps us upright.

There is increasing scientific evidence for this view of human energy fields. For years, scientists have been able to detect the energy emitted by the body by measuring skin potentials. In order to measure the electrical output of various organs, researchers place electrodes on the skin. To measure the electrical output of the brain, for example, electrodes are placed on the forehead and the scalp in the cerebral area. Similarly, the electrocardiogram measures the electrical output of the heart through electrodes placed on the skin of the chest wall; the polygraph, or lie detector, measures the changes in the electrical potential of the skin, or the galvanic skin resistance. In all these cases, we are not sure exactly what is being measured, but we do know that we are

1

measuring a form of radiation; we would not be able to measure it if it were not radiant, or electromagnetic, energy. But because all these measurements are taken using skin potentials, we are not really accurately measuring the output of the organism itself; we get interference from the skin that lies between our instruments and the organ whose output is being measured.

We now have a better method for measuring the electromagnetic output of the body. Instead of using skin potentials, we can measure the electromagnetic forces around the body directly. This has to be done under special conditions, with extremely sensitive instruments. Originally, this type of measurement was done in a shielded room, so that all the electromagnetic "noise" from such sources as the electrical equipment in the building, power lines in the street, and atmospheric disturbances would be filtered out. The instrument used to take these very sensitive measurements is known as the Super Conducting Quantum Interference Device (SQUID). Originally, the SQUID was set up in a special shielded room twenty feet underground at the Massachusetts Institute of Technology. However, over the last several years, the device has been improved to the point that for some purposes it does not need to be shielded anymore, although it is of course still preferable to use such a device in a place where there is little electrical interference.

This electromagnetic output of the body is measured in a unit of magnetism known as the *gauss*. Of course, the earth itself radiates electromagnetic energy. Every particle on earth, even though it may appear solid and stationary to us, has continual activity taking place within it; it looks solid and dense because the energy is of high frequency and low amplitude. The electromagnetic output of the earth is, on the average, one-half gauss. By comparison, the electromagnetic output of the human body is one-billionth of one-half gauss. This very tiny output can be measured by the SQUID, so you can see what an extremely sensitive instrument it is.

By measuring skin potentials, scientists have found that there are both alternating currents and direct currents coming from the body. Such currents arise from the migration of electrically charged particles, or ions, in the body tissues and fluids. These AC and DC currents give rise to corresponding magnetic fields. At present, there is only one system of the human body from which an electromagnetic output has not been measured: the blood system. Interestingly, this is consistent with what I have observed about the blood system, which I like to compare to a system of freeways, roads, and side streets, with the blood itself like a trucking company that needs to have its trucks loaded and unloaded so that the ingredients can be distributed to the tissues and the organs. Of course, the trucks themselves might have electrical components, but as long as they are not interacting with each other, they would not give out a radiation sufficient to measure. I am not sure that the blood does not have some electrical output of its own, arising from what is happening within the blood system itself. But if this output does exist, it has not been measured, at least not with the SQUID.

Modern medicine loves to take blood samples from patients to diagnose what is wrong with them. If we think of the blood system as a trucking company, we can see the fallacy in this approach. The nutrients and other substances found in the blood are not of primary importance; what matters is whether there is a crew at the other end to load and unload the trucks when they arrive at their destination. We shall later examine in some detail this area of assimilation.

Besides the energy outputs that have been measured outside the body, there are other subtle forces acting within the body that are not yet understood by science. The Soviet researcher Dr. Alexander Dubrov has found that during mitosis, or the splitting of cells, there is photon radiation from the cells. As you know, photons are particle waves of light. This radiation produces a dim glow, which we might call *bioluminescence*. The photon emissions produced by the cells in our bodies are in the ultraviolet frequencies, beyond what we know as the *visible spectrum*. All the trillions of cells in our bodies are emitting such photons, from one to another. This emission does not stop at the skin's surface, for the skin is also made up of cells.

Perhaps this discovery helps us to understand some of the ancient references to light in the sacred texts. The Christian Scriptures say, "You are light," and "If therefore thine eye be single, thy whole body shall be full of light."\* The meaning of that fascinating statement may not be purely symbolic or philosophical. In Egyptian religion, a related image, the so-called eye of Horus, has been looked upon as the eye symbolizing health.

But what is meant by the "single" eye? As long as we see positive and negative as two separate things, there is no light. If you have a positive energy field and a negative energy field and they do not merge, there is no current. So, if you still see something out of your right eye that is different from what you see with your left eye, there is an unbalanced condition. You are not perceiving things in their wholeness, so you are not in a healthy state.

We know that in the human body, fluids are suspended in crystals as

\*Luke 11:34.

colloidal cells, or crystalline substances. In another series of Soviet experiments, replicated thousands of times, researchers put single cells in each of two glass test tubes. They first measured the electronic potential of each cell and its biochemical composition. The two test tubes were then placed next to each other, and nothing happened. The experimenters next injected into one of the test tubes substances that would disturb the physiological state of the single cell so that it would become different electronically and biochemically from the other, making it in effect a diseased cell. As long as the cells were in the glass test tubes, nothing happened; the diseased cell continued to be diseased, and the healthy cell continued to be healthy. The scientists then put a quartz field between the cells (actually they put the cells in quartz test tubes). Immediately, they reported, there was what they called a "mirror-image" effect. Within seconds, the healthy cells started to show symptoms similar to those of the diseased cells. Dubrov and his colleagues were able to measure at that time ultraviolet photon transference from one cell to the other. We know, then, that the crystalline part of our cellular structure is emitting photons in the ultraviolet wavelengths.

Dubrov's researchers have observed that during mitosis, the cell emits not only light but also very high frequency sound. They found that it is possible to measure such ultrasonic sound within the body. Wherever there is light, then, there is at the same time also sound. Of course, such sound goes beyond the frequencies that we can hear. Eventually, we will be able to hear the sounds of our body by amplifying and translating them so that they become perceptible to our senses, and we may then be able to diagnose those signals as one means of detecting illness.

Knowledge that was once thought esoteric is now becoming exoteric; it is becoming scientific knowledge. I believe that within the next five or ten years, you may well be able to step into an instrument, be surrounded by an electrostatic field, and immediately see a display on screens of what is happening in your body—in living color—and you will see or hear the sound of your own body. If this output can be amplified and made visible and audible to us, diagnostics will become much easier because, as we shall see later on, it is possible to tell a great deal about the state of a person's health from the patterns of emanation and absorption in his or her energy fields.

## Educating the Senses

If we realize that the human body is surrounded by energy fields that can be detected by sensitive instruments like the SQUID, we will have a better understanding of what is meant by the aura. For many people, the aura has acquired a metaphysical meaning, and it is often felt that the aura is not "really there" or that it can be seen only by very highly developed, sensitive, spiritual beings. This is a fallacy. What prevents you from seeing the aura is the fact that your eyesight is not properly educated. If you start educating your eyes, which you will learn to do in Chapter 4, you will have a greater ability to perceive the activity taking place in so-called material objects. I have seen people who are absolutely nonspiritual develop their physical vision properly and learn to see energy fields around others. I must emphasize that with proper training of your eyesight, you can observe energy fields emanating not only from the human body but also from all material substances, including plants and inanimate matter. It is not an insult to the higher species to say that a plant or a rock can have an energy field. The human body is made up of exactly the same materials as animals, vegetables, and minerals. All the elements in our bodies are the same as elements that can be found in the crust and the atmosphere of the earth. The only difference is that we have a higher level of activity within our bodies that gives us a higher energy input and output, and therefore we have a higher level of consciousness. When you expand your energy, you automatically go beyond the denser state, and things become subtler, clearer, and easier to perceive with the senses.

We might make an analogy between two substances, such as water and molasses. Both are fluids, but the molasses is thick, dense, and practically opaque, whereas water is free and clear and flowing. The same thing is true of the human body in relation to the rest of the world; we seem to be more flexible, more expandable, and therefore we have a capacity for higher consciousness. We are able to radiate out more and farther, and we are correspondingly more sensitive to things farther beyond our own beings.

Some esoteric writers proclaim that in order to perceive what we call God, the universal, the environment beyond the human environment, one has to have an extra sense. We have enough trouble with the five senses we've got, so let's not make it more difficult by adding another one to the list. You do not have to be psychic, as every book on aura seems to tell you, in order to see the energy fields around human beings. So, get away from the idea that you have to be a special person to do it.

We are living in a three-dimensional world, and beyond our three-dimensional world, there exists a multidimensional world, which we call the universe. When we speak of certain energy fields as we have measured them on planet Earth, we have to realize that is only how we have perceived them in the human environment, in Earth's environment, and in our own solar system. Beyond that we really do not yet know in what form the energy occurs. Some people often actually perceive something from those planes beyond the human environment, our planet's environment, our solar system, and even our galaxy. This experience is multidimensional, and it is impossible to recount such experiences in three-dimensional language.

But do not get the mistaken idea that you do not use your five senses for such perception. Your five senses are the receptors for any visual, auditory, tactile, olfactory, and gustatory images that you perceive. No matter what forms such images may represent on a multidimensional plane, once these images have been perceived by the senses of the physical body, they are translated into physiological events in this three-dimensional world.

Although we are limited to our five senses, they can be greatly expanded and made much more sensitive. We are capable of becoming hyperaesthetic, or hypersensitive, through our five senses. The hyperaesthetic state expands our capacity to tune in and enables us to go beyond our own immediate environment. Note the similarity between "in tune with" and "intuitive." This is not a mysterious state beyond our understanding; it can be translated into the physical because we use our physical bodies and our senses for it.

Such hyperaesthetic states can be evoked by hypnotic suggestion. Under normal circumstances, a person might not be able to perceive a certain stimulus with his or her senses, but through hypnosis it is possible to increase the sensitivity of his/her perception to a higher level. In one experiment, for example, a subject could read a book held five feet in front of him; but if it was held at a much greater distance away, he could no longer read it. This subject was then hypnotized and given special opaque glasses that had mirrors on the inside of the glass, so that he could look in the mirrors and see what was happening behind him. The book was then held twenty feet behind him, and he could read it under hypnosis. His visual acuity had been heightened beyond the normal range of perception; his senses had been brought to the hyperaesthetic state. We are now finding that if a person has the proper motivation, the same sorts of feats can be performed without hypnosis.

Such expanded sense perception, then, is physical; it is not information that is obtained psychically. Originally, the Greek word *psyche* meant "soul." Later it came to mean "mind" because, since we really do not know what soul is, it was easier to refer to mind. So, we started referring to everything mental as part of the psyche. But the broader definition of psyche as soul is actually more accurate. We say, "All of my body is in my mind, but not all of my mind is in my body." The body is like an egg yolk floating in the cosmic egg white, which contains our individual minds, and the cosmos itself is the shell. That is, the mind or psyche operates as much outside as inside the body. (As distinguished from mind, the brain is the body's computer, which perceives, directs, and activates all the different transistors, tubes, and wires that we call our physiological organs.)

## A New Look at Miracles

I recently made a trip to Europe specifically to investigate stories about some of the Christian saints. One of the saints who particularly fascinated me was the medieval Saint Nicholas of Fluë, who was a great historical figure from Switzerland and thanks to whom that country was able to retain its neutral status and not get involved in wars. I visited the area where Nicholas had lived and talked with the pastor of the local church. To the people there, the stories about Saint Nicholas were familiar historical fact.

This Nicholas was married and had ten children, so we can hardly say he lived an ascetic life. But after a certain time, with the consent of his wife, he left his family and went into the woods, where he lived for some years. There he began to eat less and less food, until finally he stopped eating and drinking altogether. He lived on for nineteen and a half years after that with no intake of food. Of course, this statement is not quite accurate because the body cannot survive without nourishment. But as we shall see later, it was a different kind of nourishment that sustained Saint Nicholas.

When I visited Assisi in Italy on the same trip, I was very fortunate to be allowed to visit the rooms that served as a virtual prison for Joseph of Cupertino (1603–1663), who is called the "flying friar." Hanging in these rooms there are pictures, which have never been seen by the public, showing Saint Joseph levitating. It was because he did such strange things at strange times that the authorities tried to hide him; he was kept locked up in his rooms underneath the church in Assisi. He lived there for years and ate and drank hardly anything, but he levitated all the time. Old church documents tell the story of how one day a huge iron cross had to be put on top of the steeple of the church, and several men were trying to get this cross up but could not do it. Saint

Joseph was sent for. He looked at the cross and said, "Oh, that's nothing," grabbed the cross, levitated with it, and put it on top of the steeple all by himself.

I heard stories about Joseph of Cupertino from a Franciscan friar who told me that documentation of these things had been unearthed from the Vatican archives. Through this friar's account, I gained much better insight into the stories of the saint that removed them from the realm of myth and superstition.

Interestingly, Saint Joseph of Cupertino did not have a crucifix or an image of the baby Jesus where he said his prayers; instead, he had a statue of Mary as a baby. He was obviously very much aware of the feminine intuitive capacities, and he took the baby Mary as his inspiration.

Although Saint Joseph may have overdone it a bit, he was not the only saint who was able to levitate. Actually, all of us levitate, although we do not necessarily recognize it as such because we think that in levitation the actual physical body should leave the ground. Let us say you get up in the morning feeling depressed and grouchy. Your energy is like a little packet of lead. If you weigh 150 pounds, you have a gravitational pull of 150 pounds, all centered in one place, and you make indentations in the ground. But when you get up in the morning feeling excited about a project you are going to work on or about the people you are going to be with, you float through the house like a butterfly. What has happened? Your energy has expanded over a much greater area; it fills the whole room now, so your gravitational pull is distributed over a much greater area, and in reality you are levitating.

In Assisi, I also heard a great deal, of course, about St. Francis. I was particularly interested to hear about the Japanese who would come to Assisi; these Japanese were non-Catholics, perhaps Buddhist or Shinto. They knew none of the Christian mythology surrounding the renowned saint. These people were merely tourists. But when they heard the stories about Saint Francis of Assisi and how he communicated with the animals and the plants, they would immediately understand the significance of these stories because through their own religious traditions, they would become very involved with the meditative process and would get in touch with the feelings associated with the stories of the saint.

It is obvious that the miracles of the Catholic saints have very little to do with Catholicism per se. Rather, they show what happens when we get in tune with the energies of our environment—not just the physical environment, but all the levels of energies that surround us. Our own personal belief systems often get in the way of true knowledge, just as the imagery of Catholicism may enhance or impede our acceptance of the stories of the saints, depending on what our own belief systems are.

What are we to make of these stories of people who can live for years and years without eating and drinking? I know from personal experience that it is possible to live with very little food. For thirty-three years, I lived on three meals a week and sometimes have been able to sustain my body for weeks with no food at all, without consciously or intentionally being on a fast.

Theresa Neumann (1898–1962) was under medical supervision as well as under observation by the Catholic church for some thirty-five years. On Fridays, she would eat a little holy wafer when she took Communion, and that was reportedly the only food she took in during all those decades. I know such things are possible because they have been done by a number of individuals, including myself.

What is really going on, then, when people are able to live without food? In what follows, I will share with you some of my own ideas about this phenomenon.

## Light as a Nutrient

I am eating all the time, even when I am not taking in food, although not in the same way that one would usually call eating.

I had the chance sometime ago to talk with John Ott, the author of the book *Health and Light.* * He was the man who was originally contracted by Walt Disney to make time-lapse photographs of plants. He would begin, for example, with the bud of a fruit tree and film it for a full year, to show its development from the bud into a flower, from the flower into a fruit, until the fruit was completely ripe. He told me that when he did this with an apple he was very successful. But then he tried doing it with the same lighting with a pomegranate, and it did not work. His whole year's work was ruined because he was filming with the same light and the pomegranate just did not want to grow. He then began to notice the effect of light on human bodies, as well as on the animals who were also in that environment. He has since set up the Institute of Light Research in Florida and is discovering the amazing influence that light has on us.

Sources tell us that the pineal gland takes in light and even that some

*John N. Ott, *Health and Light: The Effects of Natural and Artificial Light on Man and Other Living Things* (Old Greenwich, Conn.: Devin-Adair, Co., 1973).

reptiles see only by their pineal gland, not by their eyes at all. John Ott shares with me the idea that we human beings are very similar to plants in certain respects. Plants use the light from the sun, which interacts with their chlorophyll, to manufacture their own food. We are higher up on the food chain, but all the nutrients we eat can ultimately be traced to plant life and to the energy that comes from the sun.

Now, why should we have to go through all these middlemen when we can get our energy directly from the wholesaler if we human beings, like plants, use light as a nutrient and a source of energy? (This is not to say, of course, that we photosynthesize like plants.)

How can it be possible for us to live on light? In energy fields, when we go beyond the atomic level, we get to the electromagnetic level. Beyond that is the paramagnetic, which is different from earth magnetism, where we see that positive attracts negative, that is, that opposites attract. Rather, in paramagnetic fields, like attracts like, so that if we radiate out a certain frequency of energy with a certain amplitude, this will attract energy of the same frequency and amplitude. If we are radiating energy from our bodies, we thereby attract from the environment an equal particle of the same frequency and the same amplitude.

We have already seen not only that there is intuitive, psychic evidence that the human being radiates photons but also that such radiation has been observed experimentally. The brightness of this light, or photon radiation, is determined by the amplitude of the radiation. The higher the degree of excitement, the higher the amplitude and the brighter the emanation. Our consciousness is not aware of our relationship to all these particles we attract from our environment, but once we understand the principles involved, it is not so strange that we could feed ourselves in that manner.

It is very distressing to think that we in the Western world, particularly the United States, who have 5 percent of the total population of the world, have taken 50 percent of the earth's resources and that this is still the most malnourished country in the world. Because of our materialistic ideas, we have not been able to take from the environment those ingredients that can keep us alive and free of disease.

The high energy output that surrounds the human being is not only a means by which we nourish ourselves by attracting other energy of the same frequency and amplitude; it is also a means of protecting ourselves because nothing from a lower energy field can enter a higher energy field (because the higher energy will disintegrate the lower).

However, we must be careful not to deceive ourselves when we think of this light emanation as a means of protection. I have often heard people say, "I put light around me every day; that should protect me."

But remember that creating an image in the conscious imagination is quite different from creating the energy itself and thereby producing that light. *Thinking* light around you does not make light. In fact, when you think light, if you keep thinking and looking for that light, you are occupying your cerebral cortex; and when the cerebral cortex is occupied with the thinking process, it cannot create an outward flow of energy. Therefore, a lot of people who think a lot, who constantly worry, "Should I, or shouldn't I?" or "Maybe, maybe not"—that is, people who engage in the kinds of mental activity generally associated with beta brain waves—have been known to get tension headaches and migraines. They also have poor blood circulation because in order to think, you have to have energy; and in order to have energy in the brain, you need oxygen and glucose for fuel; and these have to be brought in by the blood, the trucking company. So if you get all that thinking going, the blood is occupied with bringing whole truckloads of fuel to the brain. As a result, you do not get it to your hands, to your feet, or through your body; and you have poor circulation, cold hands, and cold feet.

Perhaps it sounds a little farfetched to say that too much attachment to thinking can cause such physical problems. However, clinical medical experience has borne out these observations. To overcome the symptomatic results of excessive cerebral blood flow, the Menninger Foundation, with special temperature biofeedback training techniques, helps people learn to divert the excessive blood flow from the cerebral area back to the peripheral parts of the circulatory system, such as the hands and the feet. This is actually nothing more than learning to make the head cool and the hands and feet warm, to bring the blood away in a nonthinking process, in a passive, nonvolitional way. Such techniques are now being used successfully all over the country in the treatment of migraine and tension headaches.

I am not saying that all thinking is bad. Thinking goes on in the unconscious as well as in the conscious mind. The unconscious mind has as much selectivity and discrimination as the conscious mind, and therefore, a great deal of unconscious activity could also be called thinking. The kind of thinking process that can lead to problems is one in which we attach ourselves to the problem, to the thought itself, and thereby hold onto the problem rather than release the energy and the emotion associated with it. The brain needs nourishment for this kind of activity, to hold the thought there, to imprison it, and the blood therefore flows to the cerebral area.

What I call *decisive thinking* is quite the opposite, for it is a release of energy. As soon as one decides, one releases. Often, we don't really look for solutions when we are involved in problem solving; we claim we do, but we actually attach ourselves to the problem. That is what causes the pressure in the head, the worry, and the physiological disturbances. But when thinking leads to release, often through unconscious processes, the physiological vicious circle does not have a chance to get started.

This should explain why consciously putting light around yourself might not necessarily be helpful to you at all. There are methods for putting this light energy around you, and the best method is, of course, to have a normal, regulated function of all the organs in your body, which means that all the chakras, or subtle energy centers, have to be operating at full capacity. Let us now see how these chakras are involved in the energy output of the human organism.

## A Practical View of the Chakras

There is a great deal of misunderstanding about the chakras. As with so many metaphysical systems, it is difficult to resolve the different modes of expression used to describe the chakra system. When I discuss the chakras, therefore, I am only sharing what I have observed in the thirty-five years that I have been able to see the chakras and their energy fields and what they do in the body. I am not really so interested in the philosophical aspects; rather, I prefer to focus on the practical applications of this knowledge. I see too many people walking around absorbed in philosophy, with their eyes on the sky, and it is obvious that they are diseased, that they have all kinds of physiological problems. They are starry-eyed but slow-bodied. That makes very little sense to me; if our knowledge cannot be practical, it has little value. (This is not to deny the value of the spiritual side of life. But one cannot be spiritual without the proper direction of mind and without the proper physical vehicle through which the spirit can operate.)

According to people who can perceive these things, the body appears to have thirteen subtle energy centers called *chakras. Chakra* is the Sanskrit word for wheel; the word was chosen because those who are able to observe the chakras, by looking through the aura, see them in cross section as fast moving vortices of energy containing colors. Six of the chakras are minor in their activities, and seven are major. All seven major chakras except one interrelate with the endocrine system. Remember, however, that when I mention an endocrine gland connected with a particular chakra, I am referring, not to the chakra itself, but rather to the organ that is influenced by that energy field.

The chakras should be thought of as dynamos, dynamic centers through which the energy is distributed. This energy is distributed from the chakras as it comes into the body as well as when it goes out of the body; there is a capacity for transmission as well as for reception. The chakras are the centers that make the aura brighter and brighter or dimmer and dimmer, depending on their activity.

Each of the chakras vibrates at a characteristic frequency as it transmits energy. The energy pattern around each chakra is viewed as a vortex predominantly of a certain color, which corresponds to the frequency at which that chakra is vibrating. Similarly, each chakra is associated with a musical tone that also corresponds to the frequency of its basic vibration.

When a chakra is operating in a balanced manner, the color surrounding it will be very pale and will be the pure color of that chakra. The pale color indicates that the energy transmitted by the chakra is fine and subtle. If a chakra is not properly transmitting the energy that comes into it, the color will have a dense, dark outflow that will be apparent in the aura surrounding the chakra.

In my earlier book *Voluntary Controls,* I discussed at some length the characteristics of each of the chakras. In brief, each chakra has an external, physical counterpart in one of the seven major glands of the body. Each chakra has a characteristic color and frequency of vibration associated with the quality of the energy it is concerned with. Table 1 lists the chakras, their locations, their associated organs, and their characteristic colors and energy functions. (In Appendix B, you will find a more complete set of tables summarizing the activities and attributes of the chakras.)

The colors of the chakras are not in rainbow order; that is, the sequence of colors in the chakras, from lowest to highest, is not in the order of the spectrum. When we realize that each of the chakras resonates with a certain color, sound, and frequency, it is easier to understand how color and sound can have a therapeutic effect; they can help to stimulate and balance the activity of particular chakras. In *Voluntary Controls,* I outlined a series of chakra exercises that enable people to check the function of each chakra through meditation and color breathing. At the Veterans Hospital in Topeka, Kansas, psychotic patients were taught to do the chakra exercises every day. Through these exercises, they were able to become calmer, and their creativity was enhanced. So the chakra exercises can be useful not only in monitoring our physiological functioning but also to regulate our mental functioning.

We know that there are psychosomatic diseases. But there are somatopsychic diseases as well. That is, when your body does not operate

**TABLE 1: CHARACTERISTICS OF THE CHAKRAS**

| Chakra | Spinal Location | Organ | Color | Energy |
|---|---|---|---|---|
| Root or sacral | 4th sacral vertebra | Gonads | Red orange | Life promoting |
| Spleen | 1st lumbar vertebra | Spleen | Pink | Reserve (love) |
| Solar plexus | 8th thoracic vertebra | Adrenals | Green | Life preserving |
| Heart | 1st thoracic vertebra | Thymus | Gold | Mental (consciousness) |
| Throat | 3rd cervical vertebra | Thyroid | Blue | Expressive |
| Brow | 1st cervical vertebra | Pituitary | Indigo | Synthesizing |
| Crown | None | Pineal | Pale purple | Integration |

properly, you cannot do anything with it, no matter how powerful your mind is and how much you perceive with it, if your mind does not have the instrument through which to express its perceptions. You are like the sculptor who has a fantastic image of a statue in his mind but who does not have the clay or rock to chisel it out of: The mental image does not do anybody any good.

## Energy Transformation Through the Chakras

With our review of the function of the chakras in mind, let us return to the question of how we can nourish ourselves on pure energy, on light. We shall see in Chapter 2 that just as there is an output of energy from the body, there is also an input, which is called the *ray*. The ray takes the form of light, and the color of that light remains the same for each individual throughout his lifetime.

According to my personal observation, this light, or current, which I have also called the *ray*, enters the body through the crown chakra, which is associated with the pineal gland. At this point, the energy is pure light; but as it moves down to the brow chakra, which is associated with the pituitary gland, it is broken down into seven different qualities. The pituitary functions as a prism and breaks down the light the same way a prism breaks white light into a spectrum. The pituitary refracts the light and distributes it through the body by way of the various chakras. The pituitary is known as the *master gland* because of its role in regulating the function of the body through its hormonal secretions. As a subtle energy center, the pituitary, or brow, chakra plays a similar role in regulating and distributing energy. When the energy returns back up through the chakras after it has been distributed to and utilized by the various organs and systems of the body, the brow, or pituitary, chakra functions as the synthesizer, integrating the component energies once again into pure white light.

After the light has been broken down into seven different qualities by the brow chakra, it moves down to the throat chakra, which is associated with the thyroid gland. Here is the first place where the light starts to become denser so that it can interact with the body chemistry, and as it moves down through the subtle energy centers (the chakras), it becomes progressively denser still. At the throat chakra, the seven qualities are divided into three groups: three qualities on the right, the male, creative side, which deal with anabolism, the process of building up, whereby new substances or chemistries or forms of substances are created; three qualities on the left, the feminine, receptive side, which deal with catabolism, the process of breaking down substances, taking them out of the form in which they entered; and one quality in the middle, the catalyst, which brings anabolism and catabolism together in the total process of metabolism. These qualities of energy are used to nourish the various systems of the body, with each chakra drawing out the energy it requires.

I should make it clear that when I talk about energy transformations in this manner, I am making a symbolic statement about what I actually observe. When I perceive multidimensional planes of consciousness and energy fields, no matter how these things may occur objectively, in order for me to experience them with my senses and express what I experience, they have to be put into some symbolic form, and it is in this form that I observe these occurrences. I am explaining subtle, nonphysical, nonvisible forces in terms of concepts that can be communicated to others. When I see the light entering the head, I can really see it being bent by the pituitary functioning as a prism, and I can really see seven main colors occurring after the light is refracted. These colors represent different levels of energies, and because consciousness is a quality of energy, I associate different levels of consciousness with these energy levels. Of course, these phenomena have not been verified in scientific laboratories; I am merely reporting the way I actually perceive occurrences that are not generally considered capable of being perceived because they are multidimensional in nature.

To return to the chakras, the energy moves down from the throat to the heart chakra, the seat of consciousness. It is at this chakra that the light undergoes a transformation into fire, a somewhat denser energy form. Conversely, when energy moves up through the chakras, it is at the heart chakra that denser energies are converted once again into light. Balanced at the pivotal point in the center of the seven chakras, the heart is the cauldron in which energy is transmuted, in which lower energies are purified into higher, and higher energies are rendered denser so that they can nourish the physical body.

The heart chakra is associated with the thymus gland, which regulates the lymphatic system of the body and hence governs our immunological defenses. This mysterious gland, we are told by medical authorities, atrophies after the age of thirteen. This is considered normal. How can we call an atrophying gland normal? Every part of our bodies has a function. Is it not more likely that we are failing to utilize the thymus for the function for which it was intended? I consider it no surprise that in our society the thymus gland should atrophy at the age of thirteen, because it is at about that age that young people are launched into adulthood, that they are told they must start worrying about how they will make a living when they grow up, what kind of a person they are going to marry, and so on. Rather than make our young people aware of mental and spiritual survival, our culture emphasizes mere physical survival; and from their early teens on, it is their physical survival that is emphasized at the expense of their mental and spiritual development. The heart chakra is the seat of consciousness; little wonder then that the gland with which it is intimately associated should begin to atrophy at the point when we begin to neglect the development of the consciousness! No wonder, either, that we have such low resistance through our lymphatic system that we are perpetually subject to colds and flu, for it is this neglected thymus gland that should be giving us the protection we lack.

With its transmutation into denser form at the heart chakra, the energy moves down and activates the adrenal glands at the solar plexus chakra, then on to the spleen, pancreas, and liver at the spleen chakra. These three organs begin the filtering operation, removing the waste material created in the burning process. Finally, the energy, in its densest form, reaches the gonadal system at the root chakra, which I like to compare to a butane tank with a pilot light on it because the density of the energy here is concentrated like liquid oxygen and the energy is released very slowly unless it is activated.

As I have already said, the reverse process also takes place. Once the energy has provided nourishment, it is released out of its physical and chemical state, and it becomes subtler and subtler, until finally it once again gets to the heart chakra, the cauldron, which acts now as a refinery, transmuting fire into light; the energy becomes subtle substance once again, and finally, it comes out of the pineal.

I do not mean this description to be taken in a metaphysical sense. I am talking literally about energy conversions and changes in energy states. Of course, this transformation cannot yet be proved scientifically. Nevertheless, this is what I have observed in human energies, and I feel fortunate to be able to see these energies moving and thereby, after years of observation, to get some idea of what is going on. This is the process I have observed: the transmutation of light to fire to substance and the transmutation of substance to fire to light.

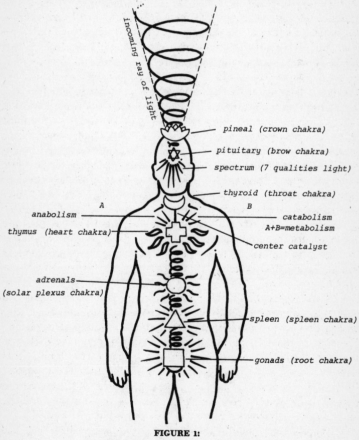

**FIGURE 1:**
**THE TRANSMUTATION OF ENERGIES**

## Energy Flow and Health

As the preceding discussion indicates, it is obvious that for an optimal utilization of energy, it is desirable for all the chakras, or human energy centers, to be functioning in a balanced, fully operative manner because the chakras, through their interrelation and interaction with all the endocrine glands, maintain normal function of all the body's organs. If one of the chakras slows down in its actions, if it is in a state of inertia, the energy flow is impeded and organs will begin to show signs of illness.

We must remember that the chakras are never completely blocked or closed. I sometimes hear some psychics say to people, "Oh, dear, your throat chakra is closed," to which I am tempted to reply, "Well, when's the funeral?" If one of the chakras were really closed, you would be dead. We can think of the spinal cord, which contains six of the seven chakras, as a pipe in which there are placed at intervals very fast-moving pinwheels that move the energy from one place to another through the whole canal. If any one of these dynamos stops, there is no way the energy can flow through, and you will not be able to exist.

If unimpeded energy flow through the chakras is the key to optimal health, it is obvious that attitudes and fears and anxieties that impede the flow can be just as damaging as actual physical injury to an organ. One area in which the destructive effect of mistaken ideas and emotions is very apparent is in the misuse and repression of sexuality. Vital, physical, sexual energy is associated with the root, or sacral, chakra. If sex is experienced only in the gonads, without undergoing transformation by rising up through the chakras, the energy is kept down in the physical realm and becomes explosive. Sexual energy is the basic life-promoting energy that provides the impetus for our organism; when it moves up through the chakras, it affects every dynamo, allowing for a holistic sexual experience.

Intercourse means interacting, interrelating, in order to become one, from the smallest particle to the total being. It is a constant balancing and merging of the male and the female, the positive and the negative, the passive and the active in each of us. When sodium and potassium ions interact in the cells of our bodies, that is a sexual act, an act of intercourse, just as much as that of male and female joining together. The sodium and potassium ions, in their interaction, procreate; that is, they produce a new form of energy, a new electrical stimulus, which, in turn, activates new groups of neurons in our body.

A very high percentage of disease can be traced to repression of sexual energy. A person may be trying to be very spiritual and may repress his or her sexuality. In so doing, he/she closes off the butane tank of his/her root chakra and also shuts off his/her emotions. Such a person might look and sound spiritual, but in reality he/she is a sick person because the energy is not flowing through him/her. Moreover, when sexual energy is held back, the higher spiritual planes are affected as much as the physical because the energy can no longer be transformed into higher levels of consciousness.

What is the point, then, of denying one's sexuality? For most people, this only leads to illness on the physical, mental, and spiritual planes. We should not deny the animal side of our natures; rather, we should give up the old negative values associated with it.

"Thou shalt not commit adultery" means to me, "Thou shalt not adulterate thy energy." We must not leave unused any of the energy that we have been given. We are adulterating God when we do things without joy or involvement of the soul. Most couples are committing adultery all the time because the sex act has become a habit; there's no totality, no communion because the communion of our bodies must be a holistic communion, drawing on vital energy to achieve a oneness at the subtlest level of our beings. There must be a spontaneous oneness to achieve total communication.

In all our actions, then, there must be total soul-mind-body union. For many people, celibacy can lead to dullness and lack of spontaneity. Such people are not using their sexual energy; it piles up, and they become nonactive and unemotional. Not much spirituality is possible in such a state. No matter what you do in life, if you do not put your full being into it, you are stagnating or adulterating the energy, and therefore you cannot consider yourself whole or healthy.

Yogis who successfully abstain from sex learn to transmute the vital sexual energy by bringing it up through the chakras, transforming passion into compassion. If they are unable to bring this energy up and out through the pineal gland, the pineal and pituitary will atrophy. So, religious celibates must not suppress or deny their sexual energy; rather, they must learn to transmute it into energies that will help their spiritual development and that will maintain their bodies as healthy vehicles.

The key to the healthy utilization of energy is creative expression. The best protection against harmful influences and lower forms of energy is to radiate energy yourself. Do not hold back your capacities; be spontaneous and joyous in everything you do. Do not compare yourself with others and worry about whether your capacities are higher or lower than theirs; just do it for the sake of doing. Do not hold the energy back for fear that someone will not like what you do; just keep bringing the energy up and out. That is your best guarantee of a healthy body.

## Input and Output of the Human Energy Cell

In this brief introduction to the idea of human energy fields, it should have become clear that what we have been talking about as the measurable electromagnetic output of the human organism, the emanation, must arise from an internal source. The outflow, the human energy fields around the human body, the individualized human atmosphere is dependent on the activity that takes place within the human body. We refer to this internal activity as the *immanence*. Even though the human body is not necessarily causing this energy, it is certainly producing the emanation of the energy that has been used and activated.

Immanence is the activity that happens within. If, through healthy attitudes and balanced voluntary control, you do not interfere with the immanence, the activity of the individual cellular structure and, beyond that, the atomic and subatomic structure, then there will be a resultant radiance. We are activated by our actions; this energy emanates from us and protects us and draws in nutrients from our environment unless we interfere with it by holding back. This is why it is so important to express our energy, to keep it flowing.

Wherever there is an output, there has to be an input. Interestingly enough, the input does not change visibly within a whole life cycle. Let us take as an analogy a common light bulb. If the light that comes from the light bulb is too bright or too dim for our purposes, we can change it; we can put in a different light bulb of a higher or lower capacity. That is, we can change the output by using more or less of the available energy. But the supply of the energy does not change; the current, the input, remains constant at 115 volts. You can plug in more and more light bulbs until finally you blow the fuses. But we humans are not likely to blow the fuses of our fuse box because we are using only about 5 to 10 percent of our total energy input. We still have 95 percent to go before we will ever blow our fuses, so we do not need to be too worried about that.

In Chapter 2, we will discuss this constant input, or the ray, in detail; and in Chapter 3, we will look at the aura, which is the output of the human energy cell. We might think of the aura as a recording; if the light bulb has been switched on and the current is now flowing into the filament of the bulb, the light is actually a recording of the activity of the current that has been set free by being released from the filament. So, if we see the human body as the filament of a cosmic light bulb, we will realize that what emanates from us indicates what has been activated within the filament. That emanation becomes a tool by which we can observe what is happening in the individual.

## Human Energies and Health Maintenance

The condition of health is a regulated, balanced flow of energy through the body, which, as we have said, receives its impetus from the chakras. Moreover, there is radiant energy emitted by the body, and this radiant electromagnetic energy bears a specific relation to the location and intensity of the activity within the body. When we realize that in the final analysis our bodies are in fact made up of nothing but energy in constant transformation, it is easier to understand how subtle, nonphysical, energetic influences such as emotions and thoughts can have a direct influence on our physical functioning, just as our physical functioning can have an effect on our emotional and mental experiences. Similarly, once we understand what produces the radiant emanation from our bodies, it is clearer why this emanation should reveal something about the state of our functioning.

What may come as more of a surprise to you is that you do not need to be psychic to benefit from the information available from observing these human energy fields. The many classes I have taught have amply demonstrated that with the proper motivation, accompanied by meditation and the eye exercises I will describe in Chapter 4, people with no particular psychic gifts can learn to see the ray and the aura. This information can be of tremendous aid to people whose lives are dedicated to counseling others or to treating others for physical illness because the subtle energy fields that surround the human body can convey advance warning of problems that may not yet have manifested themselves on the physical plane, and in any case, an understanding of these energy fields can aid in a clearer perception of what is really amiss in a case of mental, emotional, or physical illness.

Looking at the human being as an energy cell also helps us understand the roles that various sorts of nutrients play in maintaining our healthy functioning. One lesson I will be repeating throughout this book is that it is not enough to have a healthy diet or to take certain vitamins and minerals and herbs; our organisms must be able to assimilate these nutrients in order for them to do us any good. In Chapter 5, I will share my understanding of this process of assimilation, of how we attract the nutrients we require from our environment, and of how this is related to the healing properties of herbs, colors, sounds, minerals, cell salts, and other therapeutic agents.

In Chapter 6 I will describe a system I have been using successfully for many years that integrates all these diverse ways of dealing with the regulation of human energies.

The purpose of this focus on health is, of course, not simply to maintain the physical body in proper functioning order, although that is a very important goal, fundamental to the higher purposes we are pursuing. It is only through the proper functioning of our physical vehicle, the body, and the balanced, integrated functioning of our emotions, which are interdependent with the physical body, that we can begin to liberate and express the energies that come through the vehicle of the mind and finally lead to a manifestation of the soul, the spirit, the total energetic essence that is you as an individualized part of the cosmos.

# 2 : Rays

In the human energy cell, the input is called the *ray,* and the output is known as the *aura.* The ray shows a person's potentials and purposes, and the aura displays his or her present and past experiences. Because each of us is unique, every ray and every aura are different, even though all rays and auras are formed from combinations of the three primary colors as expressed and blended by the seven chakras.

There are seven different rays that may be found in different combinations in different people. Before we discuss the qualities of these seven principal rays, let us examine how the ray is created.

### The Origin of the Ray

If you will recall the light bulb analogy in Chapter 1, you will remember that there is a current of electromagnetic energy that enters us through the pineal gland and is then distributed throughout the body. This current activates the body, which begins to radiate. The process is very much like switching on a lamp, which then manifests that energy current. Each of us is activated by the same energy current, but each of us therefore expresses that same current in a unique way, depending on our own different experiences.

This current is the ray, which is a metaphysical term for a purely physical phenomenon. (See Figure 2.) The incoming current looks like a vortex or cone. The ray, or current, is essentially pure white light, but it starts to change color as soon as it hits the human atmosphere in the

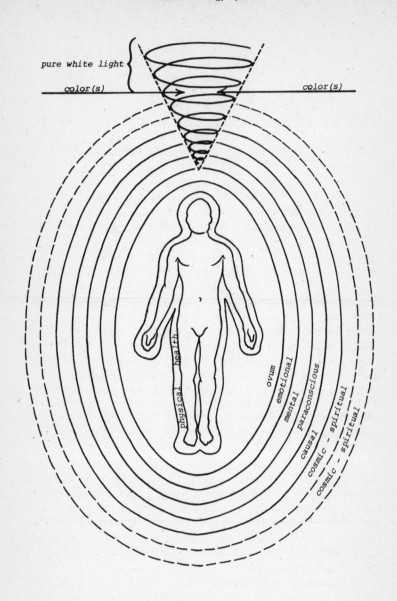

**FIGURE 2: THE RAY**

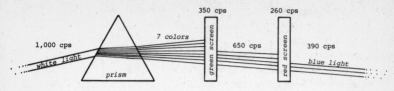

**FIGURE 3: REFRACTION OF WHITE LIGHT AND PRODUCTION OF THE RAY
BY SCREENING EFFECT OF THE AURA**

region of the causal aura. The causal aura is an emanation from the human organism, and it affects the white light of the ray. In a way, you could say that there is a rainbow effect; the density or vibration of the aura functions as a prism and refracts the light. Different frequencies are separated out, and different colors result.

Everything that your particular energy field has experienced through the ages has produced patterns in your emanation, or aura; these patterns exist as particle waves of light of varying frequencies and amplitudes. This pattern absorbs from the white light of the current all the frequencies that correspond to it, on the principle that like attracts like. What remains is everything that your energy capacity has not yet experienced.

Imagine that I have a prism and that I send a ray of white light through it. Let us assume that the combined frequencies of this light total 1,000 cycles per second (cps). The prism will refract the light into seven different colors, or qualities (see Figure 3). What frequency is present now? What was 1,000 cps when it entered the prism has been subdivided into seven different frequencies that together total 1,000 cps.

If I place a green-absorbing screen in front of the seven colored beams, what will happen? Green has a frequency of about 350 cps, so the green screen will absorb 350 cps out of the 1,000 cps. What we then have left is 650 cps. Now we put a red screen beyond the green one. Red has a frequency of approximately 260 cps, and the screen absorbs and attracts its own vibratory rate; thus, only 390 cps emerge from the red screen. Vibrating at 390 cps is the color blue. Although the incoming color was white, the color seen at the end is blue because the other colors have been filtered out (see Figure 3). Similarly, the color seen in the ray after it hits the human atmosphere is determined by the screening effect of the aura.

In Chapter 3, the origin and dynamics of the various auric fields surrounding the body will be fully discussed; at present, it is only necessary that you understand that the aura is the storehouse of your past experiences. These experiences have been translated into different frequencies of energy. When the white light current comes into contact with these energy patterns, the principle of like attracts like holds. The remaining current of unabsorbed energy represents the experiences you have not yet had. Thus, the color of this ray reveals the potentials within you that you are striving to be actualized in this lifetime.

The ray, which remains the same throughout this lifetime, shows you the tools in your toolbox. The only change that occurs in the ray is that it will become paler in hue as you use your tools. The current will look more subtle because it is more active. If you do not use these potentials, the ray remains as dense as it began, and the color will be dark. When you activate the energy it represents, the ray becomes subtler because you do not hold it back but, rather, keep it flowing in and out.

For an example, let us imagine a block of houses that are all on a 115 volt current. One house is brightly illuminated by the many lights that are shining inside, and beautiful sounds are coming from it; every little bit of that 115 volt current is being used. But in the house next door, there is just one little light glowing in the front room. Both houses have the same potentials, but one is not putting that energy to work. Similarly, having a beautiful input does not necessarily imply having a beautiful output. The aura depends on your use of the potentials inherent in that inflowing current called the ray.

Most of the time when people say they see a certain color around you, they are really seeing not your aura but your ray, which is brighter because it is the totality of all your input. Because you do not use all your input, your output is never as bright.

## The Ray in Counseling

The color of the ray can help us to perceive our purposes and to discover our inner potentials for achieving those purposes. This is an important insight because many people never understand their purpose in being alive and are never able to find deep satisfaction in their activities. We often cling to the set patterns in our lives and fail to realize that our greatest potentials or tools are going unused. I am amazed to observe the wonderful capacities in some people's input while at the same time seeing hardly anything coming out of them.

Based on my personal observation, it appears that most people are involved in pursuing the wrong goals and are trapped in inappropriate situations. They are fighting against themselves every day and thinking to themselves, "I know I shouldn't be wasting my energy on the things I'm doing, but I don't have the courage to change it." It takes great courage for someone to let go of what he/she has in order to attain a more fulfilling existence because this new life cannot be seen until the old life is sacrificed. Most people do not dare to bring out their potentials, and they keep hanging onto something with which they are completely dissatisfied. I feel that if we become aware of the dominant purpose of our lives, which is revealed by the rays we are working on, then we become much more capable of resolving our hang-ups and our problems. We are then encouraged to be what we were born to be.

Each of us has an individual function in the universal order of things. One of the most important questions people can ask themselves is: What is my purpose? It is a sad thing if they do not discover that purpose until they are very old. In my counseling work, I find it rewarding when a mother brings her just-born child to me and we can observe the baby's ray. We can learn what an infant is capable of becoming, what all its attributes and potentials are. With this knowledge, the child can be encouraged to develop desires consistent with its inborn purpose. Without such knowledge of our particular potentials and purposes, society gets a hold on us and often dictates our goals and activities, telling us that such and such an activity is most worthwhile because it will enable us to make more money or to have more power. If at a later age we finally become aware of our true purposes, we feel we have wasted a lot of time.

The ray is obviously a powerful tool in counseling; it is the main area I use in my own counseling work. Because they are not fulfilling their given potentials, many people are emotionally and physically disturbed. Once they are helped to recognize their true potentials, they can understand how they have been working against themselves.

Of course, knowing the color of the ray is only one means of beginning to fulfill individual potentials. There are many, many types of personal introspection, contemplation, and exploration that will also help us in our efforts to know ourselves. It is only through such self-knowledge that we can achieve the growth and harmony that are the purpose of life. The ray and the aura are special tools in this quest.

## Types of Rays

I have observed that there are seven principal rays and four forms in which those rays may appear. Of course, a ray can be a single color, in which case we simply refer to it as a *ray,* or a *single ray* (See "A" in Figure 4). Frequently, the ray is not a single color but is formed by a *main ray* and a *subray* (4B); such a ray might show, for example, 70 percent of one color and 30 percent of another color. When the main ray is surrounded by the subray, the subray is the one that is most active because it is open to environmental stimulation. However, even though the main ray is hidden from view, it is still potent because it expresses the majority of the energy of the current. In contrast, when the subray is in the center of the main ray (4B), it is often repressed. That is why it is often difficult to get to know people with this type of ray. You can get only so far in your acquaintance with them, and suddenly you hit an obstacle. You know there is more to them, but you cannot gain access to a part of them, the subray they have not yet activated. (And sometimes, the individual may be rather difficult to reach even when both rays are activated.)

My own ray is 70 percent pink on the inside. The subray on the outside is blue. Pink is the ray of service; it is the cosmic nursing or nourishing ray. Pink-ray people always feel compelled to serve others. It is a very highly emotional ray because it is red, which is vital energy, and white, which is all energy merged together; so, it is a life-promoting color. Surrounding the pink in my ray is blue, and blue is the color of volition, of will power or cool authority. In my case, I can get highly emotional and start to exaggerate and blow things up out of proportion because that excitable pink drives me to make sure I get the picture across. If I become emotional, I jokingly say to myself, "Uh-oh, my pink slip is showing. I left my blue head at home!" Immediately I put my blue head on, and it mellows and controls the high emotion because I become the disciplinarian, and discipline starts to direct this excitable, life-promoting energy. The blue ray, then, is actually like my voltage regulator. Yet, there are other days when I catch myself becoming authoritarian. Then I say, "Uh-oh, I have my blue head, but I'm naked, so I had better put my pink slip on." Then I have to mellow this harsh, authoritarian, dictatorial attitude with the pink ray of service and compassion.

This can give you an idea of how the qualities in the rays can be used as tools. Now, a person who had blue on the inside and pink on the outside would have trouble controlling the dramatic emotions of the

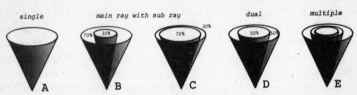

FIGURE 4: TYPES OF RAYS

pink. He/she would need to reach into his/her depths to bring the blue into action so that its radiations could calm the pink. It is, of course, possible to activate both qualities at once; then the ray becomes purplish. If it is working as an integrated energy field, using all the available potentials, then a purplish mixture or glow is seen near the blue and pink. Even though the essence of the ray itself does not change (it is still blue and pink), it works together in harmony, and you see this reflected in the aura as this integrated activity radiates forth. The two qualities are then working in unison, with balanced or equal power.

Another mode in which a ray may occur is when two rays have equal weight. When each color expresses 50 percent of the current, it is called a *dual ray* (4D). In counseling sessions with a dual-ray person, I often say to them as we begin, "You're very indecisive, aren't you?" And they look at me in astonishment. I say, "You've got poor circulation, too." They agree and ask how I know this. I explain, "You've got a dual ray, 50 percent of one and 50 percent of the other, and you never know exactly which toolbox you're going to use." It is like having a carpenter's toolbox and a plumber's toolbox, each containing a hammer that looks a little bit different from the other. Dual-ray people are constantly wondering which tool to use, so they play cosmic Ping-Pong: "Should I, or shouldn't I?" Many people with dual rays seem to be born with their sun in Libra or Gemini; that is the only correlation I have ever seen between sun signs and rays. (Needless to say, not every dual-ray person is a Gemini or a Libra.)

One more type of ray to consider is the *multiple ray* (4E), which is seen relatively rarely. It might be made up of three colors, for example, divided into 40 percent and 40 percent and 20 percent. Three different rays are occurring at once: One of the seven principal rays is a multiple ray, made up of three different colors, and there is another that is a two-colored ray. In the following analysis, these are the first and second rays, respectively.


## The Seven Rays

Let us now take a look at the seven rays. The order in which they are given here does not denote a hierarchy of importance or a sequence that is followed in any way; it is simply my system of organizing the different qualities that correlate with the colors in the incoming energy current.

In my classes, students are asked to determine which of the seven rays is their ray. They are frequently able to guess correctly simply by considering the characteristics of each ray. Of course, it is not possible for me to validate your choice visually as I would do in class. However, if you practice the exercises given in Chapter 4, you should be able to confirm the color of your ray with your own vision. There is nothing miraculous about seeing the rays, it simply takes practice.

In attempting to understand the rays, it is helpful to realize that they represent various combinations of the primary qualities in human nature. Everyone has all these qualities in varying degrees, but each of us has a unique mixture, with different emphases on the various aspects.

As I perceive and understand it, the ray of each individual is the main current of energy entering from the universe into the human being. As I mentioned in Chapter 1, the chakras are the dynamic distributing centers of the ray. We might say that the ray is the main power line from central power station, the universe, and that the chakras are auxiliary distribution centers on the main power line.

### First Ray: Electric blue, white, vermilion red
*Qualities: power, will, courage, leadership, self-reliance*

The three colors of this ray can be in harmony, but frequently one color is emphasized, and the potential balance is lost. Walking the path of this ray is like walking a razor's edge. It takes great concentration and balance to handle its power.

We can more readily understand the origin of the power in the first ray if we examine its underlying principle. The three rays in one are actually a trinity. In Christian symbolism, its equivalent is the Father, Son, and Holy Ghost. In our own beings, the trinity is the soul, the mind, and the body. We can see these three aspects in the seven chakras, correlating with the pineal, pituitary, and thyroid centers. The red ray signifies the creator God; the white ray reflects the totality of the godhead and is the Christ consciousness; the blue ray is the expression or manifestation of the creative energy. An individual working on the first ray must bring out all these qualities at once, and that is why this path is one of the most difficult. It is also quite rare.

If you could look into these people's lives, you would see that they are constantly in turmoil within themselves. They have difficulty choosing their direction. Their main characteristics are courage, will power, and self-reliance. But when the quality of power overwhelms the other aspects, they seek to conquer. This defeats their purpose of expressing the trinity because God does not need to fight or conquer.

Actually, we can say that the goal of the first ray is to merge the individual's will with God's will, to transmute the human ego with the divine ego and then express it. It takes courage to allow the two to combine because it means that the individual must face the unknown. The only place where the divine will can be found is within the seat of your own consciousness. It takes a lot of courage to enter the unknown realms of the inner self. Too many people stand in front of the mirror and see only their personal identities, rather than the unknown, divine inner self. They can perceive only the outer shell. It takes courage to drop the shell and look deep inside. This is the greatest struggle for first-ray people. Because they have power in the world, they are often the last to turn their eyes inward and find even greater powers there. Although they exercise a strict discipline over the physical and mental realms and over other people, first-ray people often lack courage when it comes to the challenges of the spiritual realm.

However, when the individual having the red, white, and blue ray achieves an integration of the three qualities, he/she becomes a leader in the highest sense of the word, by providing others with a model of behavior. There is then no power or conquest involved. Rather, the energy flows through him/her and becomes a continuum of inflowing and outflowing light. People with this ray can collect enormous energy and then express it and thus create an exemplary model of self-reliance for others to observe. However, in order to be self-reliant, one needs to sacrifice the self to the self by understanding that the self is an expression of the entire cosmos, that it is complete in itself and does not need to seek its completion externally.

In medieval times, first-ray people often became alchemists, transmuting energy into its manifested form as power. First-ray people can also become pioneers or great statesmen or even dictators. Unless their power has a spiritual goal, it can drive them to seek victory over the world. Hitler was on the first ray, as I have confirmed from personal observation of the Führer during World War II. He used his power in a negative way because he was fixated on material goals. Using the capability of the first ray to entrance or hypnotize people, Hitler was able to lead them into actions that they would not have committed under their own wills. There are many examples of dictator types who could fascinate others into following them. Although we have no actual visual proof of the fact, Rasputin and Napoleon also exemplify the first-ray type who is functioning on will power that is directed by unconscious motivations, without the higher spiritual guidance that would bring purity to their actions.

First-ray people can become confused by their power and try to make everyone else subordinate to themselves. In fact, their only true satisfaction will come from finding the ultimate reality of themselves. Their power should be used for this quest alone, but few have the courage to face this enormous goal. Instead, they choose the easier way and express their energy in physical domination.

In personal relationships, first-ray people behave in a distinctive manner. They guide and direct and are quite charismatic, with little softness in their manner. When they say no, they mean it, though they may have a certain kind of grin on their faces. They know that we often hurt what we love. There is a saying that "gentle doctors make ugly wounds." The first-ray person is not a gentle doctor when he guides. He is a rough surgeon who puts the knife to you and cuts. After you bleed, he collects the blood and pours it back into you.

First-ray people are at their best under adversity; it is then that they can test their power and leadership. When everything runs smoothly, there is nothing to challenge them. They like to tackle a tough problem and solve it quickly by taking actions that others may not even understand. They can be like pile drivers, using their enormous power to overcome difficulties or to convert you to their beliefs. Ultimately, they can transcend this forcefulness and become examples of their beliefs, rather than dictators.

A fully developed first-ray person teaches by saying to the students, "Don't come to me anymore. I have learned by doing. So if you would follow my example, stop asking me what to do. You *know* already, so begin to act." But only those who have learned to integrate the three rays and all their qualities can achieve this ideal.

The highest attainment of the first-ray individual is to move beyond human laws and social restraints and themselves to become the law; then divine will and their personal will become one. When this occurs, they can display amazing abilities. Their power over physical reality allows them to materialize and dematerialize. They have dominion over nature because they use the laws of nature effortlessly to fulfill their higher goals. Although such abilities were demonstrated by great masters such as Christ, the concept of Christ consciousness goes beyond the first ray's potentials. Christ no longer needed the power of the first ray because his spiritual awareness was so expanded that he could use another tool to fulfill his purpose—the method of nonresistance, which in the new age to come will replace the present attitude of an eye for an eye, a tooth for a tooth. Christ worked on the pure white ray; he was not involved with any of the colors anymore.

As first-ray people struggle to integrate the trinity of qualities and achieve balance, they are vulnerable to certain weaknesses. These include tyranny, self-will, pride, domination, thirst for power, and rigidity. Rigidity in the mind often makes the body rigid, so first-ray people often suffer from arthritis. Try to change their mind and you are sure to fail! When they experience defeat, degradation, and displacement, they are easily humiliated.

Despite these problems, first rays have a wonderful destiny to fulfill. When they achieve harmonious interaction among the three aspects of their beings, they embody the connection between the microcosm and the macrocosm. They personify the law of correspondences: as above, so below. When this powerful ray is integrated by the attainment of a highly spiritual awareness, it no longer appears as three distinct colors; it becomes one flowing hue, a soft lavender orchid color. This can lead to confusion when you are observing someone whom you formerly observed to be on the first ray. When the three colors blend, the individual now suddenly appears to be on the seventh ray, which is purple. However, this temporary state of affairs occurs only rarely, and the three colors are really there, although they are blended and appear for the moment to be one.

## Second Ray: Azure blue and golden yellow
### Qualities: universal love, wisdom, insight, intuition

This is the only two-colored ray among the seven rays. Basically it can be called the *messenger ray*. The blue signifies the ability to give form, and so it manifests the content of the golden yellow, which is wisdom. Thus, second-ray people who emphasize the golden yellow tend to be clairvoyants and are especially sensitive to paraconscious sources of information. If they utilize the blue more than the gold, they become teachers, religious reformers, or healers. The qualities of the second ray are love and wisdom. Wisdom is the knowledge gained when you experience something through your mind, body, and soul; then you *are* the knowledge. It is much more than an intellectual knowing; it is knowing something by being it, doing it, and living it.

How, for example, can one *know* love? We can only know what we already are. If we look within our natures, it is clear that we are a part of the whole universe, children of God or expressions of the divine spark. As this realization dawns, it is accompanied by a feeling of the love of God. People cannot have love unless it is through the love of the divine. It is that simple. We start with the source at all times, and we cannot attain the love of humanity simply through the love for our fellow humans. We have to attain it through the source, through the divine love that we carry within us, that we in fact are.

Love and wisdom are born together; thus, the Greek words *philos* (love) and *sophia* (wisdom) combine to give us *philosophy*. When there is love, there is also understanding that can embrace both the positive and the negative qualities of the loved one. When I hear someone say, "I love her/him, but I do not understand her/him," I recognize that that is a man-made love, not God-love; for one would not separate the good and bad aspects of a person's being if he/she realized that that individual is endowed with the totality of divinity and is expressing that God within to the best of his/her ability. By experiencing the divine within ourselves, we are able to love others wholly. Thus, the path to the inner knowing that is wisdom is also the way to true loving.

The golden and blue ray identifies the messengers of this universal love. These people do not care if they gain recognition or appreciation from others. Because they recognize the God within themselves, they follow an individual journey guided by the insights from their open channel to the paraconscious mind.

They combine universal love with the ability to express that love, and thus they are deeply compassionate. Empathy, not sympathy, is their attitude toward others. They take action and help to relieve the suffering in the world because they feel no separation from the rest of humanity. The second ray sees you as him/herself. Without judging your condition, he/she tries to alleviate your difficulties. The motivating impulses of second-ray people are to save, to teach, and to share love and wisdom. They are messengers who will go through fire to fulfill these impulses. In its highest expression, people on this ray are entirely selfless, nonattached, and fully aware of the unity of all life. They say, "You are me, and I am you." Any philosophy or profession that strives toward a realization of the whole human potential of giving flesh to the Word partakes of the qualities of the second ray. For example, doctors who treat the mind, body, and soul as an integral system are practicing the new age medicine under the auspices of the gold and blue ray.

Using the capabilities of the second ray, individuals can act in ways that benefit everyone. In a way, they are messiahs (meaning messengers) who bring light and the message of an unlimited universal love. This is the maximum development of the second ray. However, it takes much trial and error in life to accomplish this perfect expression. As is true for people of all categories of rays, if an individual does not realize his/her purpose, his/her life is a meaningless puzzle. If a second-ray person does not put into action what he/she knows intuitively, thereby validating it, he/she becomes dull and resentful. Stagnant pools become cesspools. Rather than loving, second-ray people can carry the most hatred and bitterness of all the rays. In such cases, they actually hate themselves because they do not understand themselves, and sadly, they beam this at everyone else in the world.

Even those who have awakened to their potentials suffer when they are unable to express them perfectly. Sentimentality and attachment, rather than love, then emerge; sensuality and passion take precedence over compassion. Such people are impractical and sometimes naïve, impulsive and unwise in their actions. You could say they have their heads in the clouds but are unable to bring what they see down to earth; they assume that abstractions and ideas are higher than the concrete, earth-based expressions of things. Isolated in their unmanifested visions, individuals on the second ray can suffer from loneliness. Often their hearts are broken because they feel alienated and misunderstood by others. Such individuals withdraw until they are martyrs. At that point, the most help someone can give them is to scold them for their self-pity. They need other people, for their creativity is expressed only when they can bring their wisdom into the world.

When individuals on the second ray express their imbalances in disease, they are prone to mental disorders, skin ailments, and dysfunctions of the liver and the pineal gland.

### Third Ray: Emerald green
*Qualities: comprehension, mental power,*
*adaptability, tact, impartiality*

The color green finds its origin in the blending of two primary colors, blue and yellow. This ray is not to be confused with the second ray, which is blue and gold, and which consists of two separate, distinct colors. Blue symbolizes will power and volition, and yellow is the color of intellect. Green-ray people give form to many creative ideas that they seed in the consciousness of others. However, they are only planters and do not stay to garden and watch the seed grow into a fruit-bearing plant. Using their excellent ability to evaluate, they choose fertile fields and know just what is needed for certain plants to grow.

I am using this analogy with plants for the particular reason that green-ray persons are the greatest lovers of nature. They feel most at home in a green, natural environment. Of course, they avoid crowds and seem aloof at times. When they enter a room, they have a cooling effect, unlike a first-ray person, who activates and thus heats the atmosphere.

The main potentials within the green-ray person are creative ideation, innovation, and inventiveness. Green-ray people are sources of ideas, but they rarely implement them. Rather, they provide impetus for the creativity of others, encouraging personal growth and the perception of the divine nature of all people. People on the third ray excel as healers of the body, mind, and spirit. They are impartial judges who love truth and quickly discern what is false. Logical, reasonable, and practical, green rays can build powerful intellects. Many great scholars, philosophers, and authors are on the third ray. They are extremely critical, but their criticism is mostly constructive and nonpunitive. In fact, some third-ray people will withhold criticism for fear of hurting others.

Because of their perceptivity and love of perfection, these people have difficulty in allowing the seeds they sow to develop as they will. Not all seeds will grow. If the green-ray person stays and watches the seeds, his/her own growth stops and he/she may even suffocate the seed. The lesson to be learned here is to become nonattached to creative efforts, to let them go and create more. Often the third-ray individual tends to be a perfectionist; fear of acting in an imperfect way then makes the individual indecisive. This ray cannot bear to make mistakes or suffer any indignity; he/she may be quite cunning in order to avoid these discomforts. There is also a possibility of becoming too judgmental and critical of oneself and of others.

Most of the green-ray people I have observed are quite introverted. They generally prefer to write what they feel and think, rather than to speak it.

Green rays are most susceptible to malfunctions of the kidneys and the pituitary gland. They may suffer from hypothyroidism, water retention, consumption, and poor circulation.

### Fourth Ray: Tawny bronze orange
Qualities: stability, harmony, rhythm, beauty, balance

The tawny bronze orange color of the fourth ray is derived from a mixture of red, the color of energy and vitality; yellow, the color of intellect; and green, the color of growth. The red and yellow blend to yield orange, the color of intuition; the more orange the ray, the more intuitive the person is. However, it is only when there is also a blending of some green, to give the ray a tawny, bronze hue, that a practical element is added to the intuitive.

More than any other type, the fourth ray wants to create harmony. To sum it up in one word, these people are *catalysts*. They have a clear intuitive knowledge of the tools in their tool kit, and they use them to find the beauty they love in others and in the world. Some become cosmic sponges, psychically absorbing everything around them, whether it is positive or negative. They like to be in the middle of everything, even to the point of meddling in other people's problems.

Usually, they have a beneficial effect and are capable of bringing peace where there is a battle of opposites occurring. That is why I envision them as being like the fulcrum of a lever. They do not empower or enlighten, but they provide the balance necessary for the other rays to act effectively.

The fourth-ray person rescues others from extremes and imbalances. People tend to confide in these orange-ray individuals, who often carry the burden of others' problems. This ray is particularly connected with the energy of the heart chakra. Until individuals attain a perfected expression of this energy, they may be quite flighty and indiscriminate about love. Sometimes, they become so eager to fulfill their ray that they try to bring harmony everywhere; they are then inconsistent in their emotions and rather unreliable and impractical.

Orange-ray people are also jacks-of-all-trades but masters of none. They have to act on the impulse of the moment, and specialization would demand too much concentration of them. Their ideas and interests vacillate from moment to moment; they need variety and would become bored if they were to continue at one specialty. They need to express themselves in beautiful ways, and so many are artists. Because their purpose makes them quite reliant on the attention of others, they tend to overdramatize and inflate emotions and situations beyond the actual facts. When they cannot play their catalytic role, they become moody and extremely depressed. This is a difficult ray to live. Even though it imbues individuals with a glow of charisma, they often fall prey to self-indulgence and conceit. At times, they will use any method to attract the attention and involvement of other people so that they can play a controlling role in life.

Orange-ray people, seeking their own balance in order to be perfect harmonizers of others, are prone to certain physical problems, including a tendency to obesity, water retention, and either hyperthyroidism or hypothyroidism.

### Fifth Ray: Lemon yellow
*Qualities: logic, accuracy, tolerance, patience*

This is the ray of the intellectual function in its purest expression. Individuals with a yellow ray love facts. Their motivation in life is to find out the answer to every question, to verify their knowledge through logic. Although their vision is narrow, this single focus helps them pierce the shadows of ignorance and discover new information. They can offer clear explanations of things, but their manner of presentation is rather dry because they fear that expressing emotion will get in the way of facts and figures. Hence, yellow-ray people have extreme difficulty in relaxing and relating to others in a spontaneous way. They are very serious and solemn; are objective about their ideas; and stimulate people with excitement about their ideas.

These are the people who know every word of the law and uphold it rigidly. Because of their tunnel vision, they are frequently unable to see the whole picture, to understand how the facts fit together. Yet they love chess or puzzles because of the intellectual challenge and the lack of emotional involvement. More materialistic than any other ray, fifth rays cannot stand criticism and are rarely involved in a quest for self-knowledge. They make excellent researchers and lawyers. In the arts, they are mainly interested in form and accuracy, rather than in inspiration.

Fifth-ray people have provided the world with precise information about our physical universe. They develop and implement the faculty of conscious, rational thought until it is razor-sharp. Because of this focus in their life purpose, they tend to suffer from inflexibility of mind and body. Thus, their main physical problems are migraine headaches, muscle spasms, and arthritis. Meditation and relaxation methods combined with visualization exercises may help them to discover other aspects of their beings and become less rigid.

It is relatively rare to find a person with a pure yellow ray; most have subrays, and so the moderating influence of the subray can be brought out through appropriate disciplines.

### Sixth Ray: Rose pink
*Qualities: one-pointedness, devotion, sacrificial love, loyalty*

The pink ray produces evangelical people. They serve others. In doing so, they are actually serving themselves and fulfilling their primary goal of teaching people to raise their consciousness. The sixth-ray person seeks to help everyone realize the angelic nature within themselves. They always have a cause to which they are totally devoted. Because they feel that they are particularly in tune with the cosmic order, they can be intolerant of the advice of others and resentful if they are misunderstood. People on this ray are capable of sacrificing their lower egos to their humanitarian goals. They are romantic, emotional, and sentimental and will martyr themselves for love of their cause.

They can give themselves totally and are the most loyal of all the rays. This is because they understand inwardly that if they are true to themselves, they are automatically true to others.

When the red component of the pink ray is dominant, these people can be fiery evangelists whose enthusiasm can lead to martyrdom. Such a lack of balance makes them masochistic and thus less effective in fulfilling their mission of love.

Sixth-ray people may try to teach in too soft a manner. There is one word in the dictionary that they do not know, and that is *no*. They hem and haw, and the best they can say is, "Well, no—but perhaps." Gullible, tender, and hesitant, pink-ray people are somewhat unsure of themselves if they must hurt you a little to heal or teach you. They cannot withstand adversity and always attempt to flow in love and harmony with others.

When these motivations and tendencies are expressed in extremes of self-sacrifice and martyrdom, pink-ray people will suffer from various kinds of abdominal problems.

### Seventh Ray: Purple
*Qualities: precision, grace, dignity, nobility, activity, integration, ritualism, designing, synthesizing*

The purple ray is a blending of red, white, and blue. Red, as mentioned previously, represents the activation of available energy, that is, power and vitality. Blue represents direction-giving power or will power. White, a blending of all colors, represents purity, truth, the all-encompassing expression of the universal source. When these colors are blended, purple results, the exact hue depending on the proportions of the colors. The more white there is, the more orchid the ray will be; the more red, the deeper purple; the more blue, the darker violet. The red, white, and blue of the first ray are not intrinsically blended; however, when a first-ray person integrates for brief periods, the resultant purple hue may be temporarily mistaken for a purple ray.

Individuals who have the purple ray are distinguished by their noble bearing. Although they are not necessarily conceited, they are misunderstood because of their regal appearance. They love ceremony and ritual and power. Many become interested in magic and have strong psychic sensitivities. However, unless they are well balanced in their own identities, they can be superstitious and victimized by lower forms of occult practices.

Purple-ray people are like suns. They need a lot of freedom to act and express themselves. If others get too close, they may be disintegrated by this powerful ray. Yet others are strongly attracted to these suns. When the sun does not respond in kind, there are difficulties in mutual understanding. Purple-ray people are frequently insecure because they are so often isolated by their acquaintances.

Another expression of the dignified quality of purple rays is a love of symmetry and formality. They grasp things as a whole and are not interested in the details of the picture. Feeling that they know more than others, purple rays would rather do it themselves and are quite self-sufficient. This, too, keeps them out of reach of many people, and they are thus slow to form relationships.

Purple rays work in fields that provide them with the opportunity to give graceful form to their holistic ideas, such as the arts, interior design, or fashion design.

Purple-ray people are motivated to maintain a noble, ceremonious, and orderly existence. Because the world in which they live is often chaotic and crude, people on the seventh ray suffer from imbalances primarily through nervous tension and disorders of the adrenal glands.

## Working with the Ray

In determining your own ray, there are a few considerations to keep in mind. First, remember that the seven rays represent qualities that are within everyone. Your ray is the particular quality that you want to learn most about in this lifetime. At first, therefore, you may actually express some of the other rays better than your own. If you had already mastered your ray, there would have been no need for you to experience it now. Unless you are quite certain that you know the color of your ray, it is best that you keep all of them in mind. As you become familiar with the qualities they embody, it will be easier to assign a ray to yourself or to others. Ultimately, by following the eye exercises described in Chapter 4, you should be able to see the rays directly, rather than infer them.

Many people do not exhibit one or the other of the seven principal rays. Instead, they have a combination of two or more of these seven rays. When such combinations are clearly defined, it is possible to understand the significance of these peoples' rays by noting the location and proportions of the various colors.

Finally, I want to caution you about observing the ray or the aura. Remember that you are looking through your own aura when you view someone else. This is why self-knowledge is so essential for anyone engaging in any type of physical, emotional, or spiritual therapy or counseling. You must be able to distinguish your own qualities and problems from those of the person you are trying to help. No one is all-seeing or perfectly self-aware. Furthermore, there may be many phenomena vibrating below or above your perceptual capacity. When

I speak with a student or a client, I always suggest that he or she take my words with a grain of salt. Each person is his/her own best judge of what is applicable to his/her own life. If you can give the fruits of your vision to others and encourage them to keep what is valuable and throw out the rest, then you have truly been of service to them.

# 3 : The Seven Auric Fields

If the ray is the input, or the current, then the aura is the output, or emanation. Whereas the ray shows what your potentials are, the aura shows what you are experiencing and what you have experienced. By understanding the patterns of the aura and mapping it out in each individual case, it is possible to make a prognosis of what a person might experience in the future if he or she uses the energies we know are available, as shown by the ray.

Everything that I will be saying about the aura has come to me in an empirical way, that is, through direct personal experience. Although I began to see these human energy fields at a very young age, I did not understand what I was seeing until much later. Over thirty-five years of observation, I have noticed that people have certain things in common—similar diseases, mental states, behavior patterns—when their auras look a certain way.

In 1971, for example, I was asked by a doctor in Vancouver, British Columbia, with whom I frequently consult, to take a look at a twenty-eight-year-old patient of his. On observing this patient, I was able to report that he had had tuberculosis in April 1963, followed by a collapsed lung—all of which the doctor was able to confirm from the patient's records. But I observed something else in the patient that I had never seen before. I remarked to the doctor, "A very interesting thing is happening in the bloodstream. It's as if I see little steel filings, looking like tiny silverfish, that are apparently attacking another, smaller, and darker particle; and after it attacks it, it sort of devours it. Every time that happens I see little ripples coming out as soon as it has been devoured. I don't know what that is." It turned out that the patient was a heroin addict and that the doctor had just placed him on methadone. The doctor suggested that what I was seeing was probably the action of the methadone on the heroin.

About three or four months later, a young man came into my counseling room, and I saw the same thing occurring in his blood! I immediately asked him, "How long have you been on methadone?" He was rather surprised, to say the least!

That is the empirical way I've learned to map out the human energy field, by seeing the same occurrence in different situations in different individuals. I am sure the mapping is not complete yet; every day, I see new things for which I do not yet have an answer. There is still a great deal to be learned about the meanings of the patterns in the aura, but I will relate some of what I have been able to learn so far.

The human atmosphere, or aura, surrounds you in every direction; although it is represented in drawings as two-dimensional, always bear in mind that it is three-dimensional. This energy field is made up of vortices that move in different directions and together make up an elliptical, or egglike, shape. Those who have read the books of Castaneda or the writings of some of the seers will recognize this description of an egg-shaped energy field. There are horizontal as well as vertical energy fields, made up of vortices within vortices within vortices.

The human aura is made up of different levels of density. As we move away from the human body, the energy fields become progressively subtler and more difficult to see. Because of this, we know considerably more about the auras closer to the body than we do about some of the subtlest ones.

We have all had the experience of observing such an energy field made up of varying layers of density, although we may not have realized it. In the familiar experience of looking at a candle flame, one can discern different levels of density as represented by different colors and degrees of subtlety. Right around the wick you will see a bluish form surrounded by a dark area that is also bluish gray. Then there is an oval shape of a golden or yellowish color, and within that yellowish oval, you can make out layers of varying degrees of subtlety. Beyond the flame itself, you can see subtler oval-shaped fields of energy, a sort of dissipating glow. The human aura, like the candle flame, is made up of progressively subtler levels of density. Let us begin by looking at the one closest to the body.

## The Physical Aura

A number of recent books have stated that the aura has been photographed. This is not exactly true. Through the use of the techniques of Kirlian photography, a small *part* of the total aura has been photographed, perhaps a fraction of an inch. The total aura may extend as far as fifteen or twenty feet, but on the average, a normal, active person will have an aura five to eight feet in diameter.

What, then, has been photographed? If you look alongside the physical body, right next to the skin, you may see an emanation of light coming out, which is called the *corona*. But between the corona and the skin, there appears to be a space, which we call the *band*, about one-eighth inch wide. This band has been photographed in Kirlian photography; in more technical terms, the band is called the *galvanic skin resistance*. The band has no color and looks like a dark gray gap or a very narrow black hole. It is neither an emanation nor an absorption; it is more like a temporary resistance to outflow. This band can be seen in the Kirlian photograph because these photographs are made by passing a high-voltage electric current through the object being photographed; there is no other source of light. The band, then, represents the resistance to the outflow of this current.

Surrounding this band of resistance, we have the first corona of the emanation. This part, which looks like a shadow form of your physical structure, is sometimes referred to in esoteric literature as the *etheric body*. In the traditional classification of the elements—earth, water, fire, and air—philosophers called the subtler substance that fills the void between these elements *ether*. This concept, in more modern terms, is once again becoming popular among scientists. It is strange that this, the densest of all the human energy fields, should be called the etheric body. I feel, rather, that the most subtle should be called the etheric, and I prefer to call this the *physical aura*. This is the aura most closely related to the physiology of the body and is the one that is used to diagnose physical disturbances. Of course, these disturbances can be seen in the other outflows as well because all the emanations are a result of the totality, but definite physiological disturbances are read in the physical aura.

In the healthy person, the physical aura extends from four inches to about eight or, rarely, twelve, inches from the body. Under normal, healthy circumstances, it is a smoky blue color, like a smoke screen around the body. Because it is the closest to the body, the physical aura is apparently closely related to the infrared frequencies, or the frequencies of heat.

Some people have claimed to see a foggy glow around a person. The first Apollo astronaut who landed on the moon was pictured in photographs as having a blue glow around him. At least one reporter said that this glow represented the discovery of a "strange energy field." Of course, that "strange energy" was there even when he was on the earth, but the airless surface of the moon made it possible for it to become visible on camera.

The physical aura is not very bright. This is in contrast with Kirlian photography, which shows it to be brilliant and colorful. What makes the corona so bright in the Kirlian photograph is that there is a Tesla coil or Van de Graaff generator connected to the instrument by which the picture is taken that generates an electrostatic field higher in voltage than the energy outside that field. The electrostatic field filters out all electrical noises and disturbances, thereby insulating the object being filmed within it; so it is therefore logical that there is a greater capacity to make an image on the photographic plate and that the image will look brighter.

Surrounding the smoky blue corona that some people call the etheric body is an energy field shaped like an egg, or an oval, that I call the *ovum*. The ovum stands about a foot or a foot and a half to two feet away from the body. It is still part of the physical aura; it is the dissipating outflow of the corona, which becomes progressively subtler the farther away it is from the body. In most cases, the ovum is of a dirty golden or ivory white color. Most people who say they have seen auras, if they were not actually seeing the ray, have seen either the corona of the physical aura or the golden-ivory ovum around people. Because this is still part of the densest of the energy fields, it is more readily visible.

In the physical aura, then, we have first the band, then the corona (which has also been called the physical aura or the etheric body), and then the ovum. The human body, surrounded by the ovum and the physical aura, resembles an egg yolk, and what surrounds the yolk, the egg white, is the other energy fields around it. The yolk floats within the energy fields that we are creating and with which we are making contact with the universe again in our subtle emanations.

The ovum resembles an egg flattened on one end, like the legendary egg of Columbus. (Columbus gave his men a riddle while on board his ship. He told them that he could make an egg stand on end. Of course, they said he could not do it, that the egg would fall over. Columbus hard-boiled an egg and pushed it down, and it stood up.) The flat end of your physical aura shows that you are integrally connected, through your energies, with the soil. Your energies are influenced by what radiates from the soil, and at the same time, you are influencing the soil you walk on.

If we could amplify the energy coming out of the body, we would see that it is made up of vortices of energy. If an organ starts to malfunction, there is not enough energy activity in it; and instead of radiating outward, it starts to absorb energy. When such absorption takes place, the emanation in the corresponding part of the physical aura begins to look dull, less blue and more silver gray; and the more it absorbs, the darker gray it will look, until eventually it would look like a black hole, or an empty space. When it is black, it represents a grave situation. Anywhere a dark spot occurs in the physical aura, you know that is where a physiological disturbance is taking place, and someone who observes the aura may see such a physiological disturbance occurring even before the person is aware of any feedback from it.

Similarly, if an organ or system becomes excessive in its action, we see a very bright spot around that area. For example, in hyperthyroidism, you would see a very bright light around the throat area. Lately, we have seen tremendously bright light around the pituitary and pineal area and around the solar plexus–adrenal system in young children who have been diagnosed as hyperkinetic or hyperactive. Unfortunately, such children are treated with drugs that suppress their high energy level. Rather than being directed to be quiet, these children should be helped to use their high energy in functional ways. It is not good to have the high energy stay around the solar plexus and around the pituitary and pineal glands. The whole body should be equally radiant, and the extra brightness in these areas shows that there is an imbalance in the system. By creatively stabilizing this energy, the child can deal with this high energy input.

Besides observing its brightness, we can also get information from the extension of the physical aura. If a person has several organs malfunctioning, so that these organs are not radiating, but absorbing energy, the size of the physical aura will become narrower, denser, more opaque because now it gives off less radiance. It does not expand so far anymore because the frequency becomes higher and the amplitude lower, and consequently, the wavelengths shorter. If the body starts to become diseased and more absorption than radiation is taking place, the ovum contracts, becomes denser, and the color is denser and more opaque, not so golden ivory as it was. So, if you saw nothing but this contraction and denseness, you would know that there is something wrong in the physical system, even though you had not yet determined exactly where the physical system is malfunctioning.

## The Emotional Aura

The next emanation I call the *emotional aura*. The emotional aura begins at the outer edge of the ovum, about one and a half feet from the body; it varies greatly in width, but on the average, it reaches out about another eight to twelve inches. Some esoteric people have called this the *astral aura* (*astral* meaning "from the stars"). It is true that this particular energy field would be stimulated by cosmic influences such as the stars, but it is also influenced by other factors, such as a person who may be affecting your emotions, that would immediately cause the emotional aura to change. The planets and the stars do have a great influence on our emotional nature, but let us not forget the lesson learned in *Voluntary Controls:* that every mental and emotional occurrence is also a physiological occurrence and so affects the radiant emanation from the physical body.

The emotional aura is one of the most difficult of the energy fields around the body. Sometimes, I have seen as many as sixty-four colors occurring at once in the emotional aura! This is because there is a lot of activity going on in the emotions all the time. The emotions are much subtler than the physical substance, and sometimes, they run ahead of the physical substance.

In the emotional aura, a multitude of different changes are constantly taking place because, even if we do not realize it, we are continually bombarded by external as well as internal stimuli, which, in turn, produce chemical changes. The secretion of hormones, for example, is based on emotional stimuli. Every thought immediately creates an emotional response, too, because emotion is *energy in motion.* The more energy that is being activated, the more reflection that takes place in the colors of the emotional aura. When the colors are excessive, we say that the person is superemotional or hyperemotional, and then the emotional state starts to have backlashes on the physical body.

Under normal circumstances, all the colors of the spectrum may be seen in the emotional aura. Where do these colors come from? Changes first take place in your physical structure. An increased or decreased state of functioning, which constitutes a transition in your physical structure, will have an effect on the chakra, or dynamo, that resonates with the outer world as well as with the inner world. This effect on the chakra will then influence the energy that you radiate; the emotional aura will show a specific color related to the specific chakra that is affected more than the others. Of course, all the chakras interact and do not really function separately, but according to the color that is seen in the emotional aura and its location in relation to the seven chakras, it is possible to tell how a certain kind of energy is being used in the organism.

The emotional aura, then, is a relatively explicit radiation indicating the action of the chakras. Of course, the colors of the chakras themselves are continually changing, just as the colors in the emotional aura are constantly shifting, but the base colors of the chakras rarely change, if at all.

Table 2 reviews the base colors of the chakras and what kinds of energies they represent.

As the table indicates, the base color of the root chakra, which is associated with the gonads, is red orange. This is the color of vital, physical energy. As we shall see, when this vital energy moves up through the chakras and is expressed at a higher level, it undergoes changes that are reflected in the colors evident in the emotional aura. The pink of the spleen chakra is the color of love. The spleen also functions as a reserve battery for the body; hence, pink also represents reserve energy. When I observe bright, clear energy fields around a person, and if my own aura is also clear and bright, the other person's body becomes translucent to my vision. Because the person is in my aura, it is as if the molecules of the body are displaced. In such cases, it is possible to see a pinkish glow around the entire nervous system; if the body becomes even more translucent, we may also see the meridians of acupuncture, which are also pinkish in color. This pink, which is associated with the subtle anatomic systems of the body, is the pink of reserve, or love, energy.

The base color of the solar plexus chakra is green, which is the color

**TABLE 2: BASE COLORS OF THE CHAKRAS**

| Chakra | Color | Type of Energy |
|---|---|---|
| Root | Red orange | Life-promoting energy, vital, physical energy |
| Spleen | Pink | Love, reserve energy |
| Solar plexus | Green | Growth and healing, life-preserving energy |
| Heart | Golden yellow; gold | Consciousness, mental energy |
| Throat | Blue | Volition, expressive energy |
| Brow | Indigo | Transitional color, synthesizing energy |
| Crown | Pale purple or orchid | Integration |

of life-preserving energy. This is the stabilizing color. As the vital energy moves up from the root chakra through the emotional plane of the solar plexus, it is preserved by being cooled down in preparation for moving into the next state, the rational and the conscious state of the heart chakra.

The heart chakra is associated with golden yellow or gold, which is the energy of consciousness, of mental energy. We have seen that energy undergoes transformations in the course of moving through the chakras and that the heart chakra is the site of the transmutation of fire into light as we move upward or light into fire as we move downward. As energies pass through the crucible of the heart chakra, they undergo transformations that are reflected in a change of color at this chakra.

The blue of the thyroid chakra is the color of will power, of volition, of expressive energy. The brow chakra has a base color of indigo, which is actually a transitional color comprising the three primary colors in the process of mixing and blending. The energy represented by this transitional color is synthesizing energy, and the pituitary gland, associated with this chakra, is, not surprisingly, called the *master gland* because it synthesizes the hormones that regulate the entire endocrine system of the body.

The purple of the crown chakra is made up of the two primary colors, red and blue, combined with white, which contains all colors. This purple or violet color is the color of integration. This chakra, associated with the pineal gland, represents the integration of positive and negative, of creation and destruction, of absorption and radiation. Energy, in the form of light, is absorbed by the pineal gland. As energy moves down through the chakras, we have seen that it is transformed from light to fire to substance; as it moves back up, it is once again transmuted from substance to fire to light. When the individual is functioning in a truly integrated manner, the violet of the crown chakra shows that the functioning of the organs and chakras is nicely balanced and blended and that there is a continuous input and outflow of energy, the input of course represented by the ray and the output by the aura.

Once we know what qualities are represented by the colors of the various chakras, we can tell what state an individual is in emotionally by interpreting the colors we see according to the types of energies they represent and where these colors are located.

The colors in the emotional aura have a definite relationship to the base colors of the chakras. In all the years I have been observing the energy fields around people, I have never seen, for example, the bright vermilion red of the root chakra occurring anywhere above the solar plexus in the emotional aura. I have often seen it below the solar plexus.

I have seen a merging of the red orange with other colors above the solar plexus, but then it becomes pink or orange or purple, violet, or indigo, but it never has the solid red orange of the base color. If you see red orange around the shoulders, there is something wrong in your observation; you are missing the color the red orange is merging with. This is a useful principle to keep in mind, a good test of the accuracy of your observation.

In a healthy state, the colors in the emotional aura are not identical to the base colors of the corresponding chakras. For example, because the base color of the solar plexus chakra is green, you might assume that if you see green around the solar plexus, it means everything is fine. But this is not so. It means that the chakra is not very active. If it is active, the colors will be in a continuous state of transformation. Green is only the base color. The more active the chakra, the smaller the base color, or axis. If the solar plexus remained green, nothing from above could come below, and nothing from below could come above. If a person has a green band only around the solar plexus area, you would say that the person was in a state of growth but was not permitting the growth to develop up from the soil, that he or she was not letting it go.

Just as the red orange is never seen above the solar plexus area, the purple of the crown chakra is very rarely seen below or at the level of the solar plexus. We see it down to the solar plexus area, but very rarely have I seen it below the solar plexus. It cannot go through the heart chakra and come out the same color in the solar plexus area below. As soon as the subtle color of purple begins to affect the heart dynamo, we see it merging into a browner, bronzer, more orange color. We are dealing with different types of forces that can intermix but that then do not retain their characteristic colors anymore.

If you see purple in the solar plexus area, either you are seeing wrong, or you are seeing an integral state between the lower energies of red orange and pink and the energies in the solar plexus area. This means that the person is emotionally integral with his own system, as well as with the outside world. When you meditate according to the methods outlined in *Voluntary Controls,* there are visible changes in the emotional aura. When you chant the second om, purple begins to appear around the solar plexus area. This represents a stabilization and integration of the upper functions with the lower. The lower energies start to pump up to the heart area, and the upper start to pump down.

Similarly, if I take the green of the solar plexus and bring it up and out through the heart chakra, it will not be the same green anymore; it will now be a yellowish green, or chartreuse, because now gold has been added to it from the heart chakra. All the colors you see above the heart chakra should have a golden sheen to them.

The only place in the emotional aura where it is healthy to see an increase in the original base color is in the heart chakra. There we see the golden orange becoming brighter and brighter with greater activity. The heart chakra is the alchemist's vessel, the cauldron in which the transmutation from fire into light and from light into fire takes place. The more that is released from below and the more that comes from above, the more activity occurs in the radiation of the golden light, and the consciousness is concomitantly expanded. The energy is so alive then that there is an arousal of consciousness that also affects the physical body; you may feel a sensation of tautness in the chest area.

## The Mental Aura

The other auras are not so complicated as the emotional aura. The next one, the *mental aura,* is a narrower band than the emotional. The emotional aura starts about one and a half feet away from the body and reaches out perhaps to a width of eight to twelve inches. The mental aura extends about ten to twelve inches in depth beyond the emotional aura. The mental aura may fluctuate somewhat; if it becomes narrower, it will become correspondingly denser.

In contrast with the variety of hues in the emotional aura, the mental aura is either two colors (the yellow of intellect and the orange of intuition) or a single golden color, a blending of the two. When it is two colors, the outer layer, which is closer to external stimuli, will respond fastest. When the yellow is on the outside, then, the person operates intellectually and does not allow the golden orange of intuition to come out. When orange is on the outside, it means that the intuitive function is stronger than the intellectual.

Because we refer to this aura as the mental aura, you might assume that this band would reflect the activity of the total mind, but it does not. The mental aura reflects only the activity of the conscious and the subconscious minds, the conscious being the intellect and the subconscious being the coordinator of physiological activity, the maker of dreams, the archives and library. When the mental aura is a single color, a golden yellow blending of the conscious and the subconscious, it means that the person is operating with synchronized conscious and subconscious minds; that is, the subconscious works with the unconscious intuition and brings it to the surface and registers it there. When the colors are blended into a single color, physiological changes will take place because voluntary control is possible. Such a person would be producing predominantly alpha brain waves because alpha is the brain wave of self-regulation.

## The Paraconscious Aura

The next aura reflects the activity of what some people have called the *superconscious mind,* or what I call the *paraconscious mind.* This is the individualized part of the universal mind, the pure, creative intuition. The paraconscious mind, besides representing your higher consciousness, also represents the universal collective consciousness. The paraconscious mind is associated with the slow brain waves of theta and delta; when these brain waves are present, there is is hypnagogic imagery that cannot be altered by conscious volition. The long wavelengths of paraconscious activity put you constantly in communication with the outer environment, including the physical environment. These wavelengths are so long that they go far beyond the physical plane of the earth. It is for this reason that your paraconscious aura is your individualized picture of what is happening in the universe, whether or not you are aware of it.

The paraconscious aura contains the same seven main colors of the chakras. The colors are not necessarily where the chakras are except for one, the gold of the heart chakra. Even though the same colors may occur in the paraconscious aura and the emotional aura, there is a difference between them. The paraconscious aura is wider in size than the emotional (approximately twelve to eighteen inches), and the colors are always lighter, more pastel. Dark colors are very rarely seen in the paraconscious aura because it is that part of the mind that is universal, the higher consciousness, and that has not been touched yet by the individual's shortcomings, by the activities of day-to-day existence.

On the paraconscious plane, you are always growing and progressing, although you may never become aware of it or learn to express your growth. The paraconscious aura is therefore never stagnant; because of the continuous action going on in this area, the colors are never dark or dense.

If you will recall the image of Pascal's communicating vessels, which I discussed in *Voluntary Controls,* you will remember that when three vessels are all open and connected to each other, fluid that is poured into one vessel will flow into and fill all three to an equal level. When pressure is put on the surface of the fluid in one of the vessels, the flow into the adjacent vessel will be blocked. In the same way, mental blockages will prevent our intuitive knowledge from flowing out of the paraconscious mind into the subconscious and the conscious minds. All our traumas are actually like a surface pressure, a suppression of the flow of information from the universal mind. So, even though you keep on moving and developing on a universal plane, you might not see any indication of it. Even though you are in constant communication with the universe at large through your paraconscious mind, you will not be aware of it unless you release the energies and avoid putting pressure on the subconscious mind. This is why the cosmic review, as a part of nightly meditation, empties out those vessels that have pressure on them and restores the intuitive flow.

Compared with the emotional aura, the paraconscious aura is much lighter, reflecting greater brilliance and intuitiveness. For the emotional aura to look like the paraconscious would mean to integrate the colors, to become more transpersonal. The most favorable state would be to have the emotional aura exactly equal to the paraconscious aura, which would mean that the person is emotionally expressing what the soul actually dictates. In such a case, the mental aura would be one integrated color, and we would see a merging of the three auras together.

Is it possible for us personally to do anything to increase the action of the paraconscious mind on the rest? If we go into theta brain waves, we become aware of what is going on in the paraconscious. There are a number of techniques being explored for voluntarily going into theta, both with the mechanical assistance of biofeedback instruments and, in meditation centers, without the use of instruments. When people learn to go into the theta brain wave at will, they become more intuitively creative.

## The Causal Aura

We know very little about the *causal aura* because it is so subtle. We might also call this the *soul emanation* because it deals with the soul essence, the individualized capacity of energy that we call the soul. This is the aura in which the ray first becomes visible because it is in this aura that all the experiences you have gone through as a soul, or capacity of energy, lead to the absorption of various frequencies and amplitudes. Out of the pure white light that is your input, what is left after it hits the prism of the causal aura is the ray you operate on, or what I have called your toolbox. If the causal aura shows what your soul essence has experienced, the ray shows all the potentials of what you have not yet experienced.

I have very rarely seen more than two (and at most three) colors in the causal aura. At first, I understood very little about the meaning of the colors in this aura; but through years of observation and of questioning of the people whose auras I have observed, I have come to some understanding of it. It is the result of the source of your being; your whole being is dependent on that substance, what we call soul. The colors represent the different qualities of energy you have experienced in what we might call *former life experiences.* When I say former life experience, I do not necessarily mean life in a human body on this planet. I'm talking about life experience as energy—in what form it may have been, I do not know. I personally believe, and I know from experience with a two-year regression research project, that there is such a thing as reincarnation and that it might be possible to go into another physical body after leaving this one. But if we look at it from the context of universal time, it would seem rather silly for us, on this one small planet Earth, to remain in just one place, in just one form of physical body, when we are surrounded by a huge galaxy, one of billions of galaxies.

When we see some white color in the causal aura, to me it means no physical existence in any form, a sort of suspended animation, pure energy activity without specific material form. This would represent a period when your beingness was pure light in essence, before it became individualized, before there was any consciousness of its own individuality. The actual colors we observe in the causal aura may represent the last stages of the person's physical appearance, the memory patterns of the ray characteristic of the person in previous life experiences.

If a person has pink in the causal aura, for example, we might assume that that person had a life of service because pink is the color of love, of service, of nursing and nourishing humankind. If there was more of a reddish glow, the person would have been something of an artist, with the inspirational energy of the red color of life force. If the color was pure yellow, I would say the person had been very scientific—and probably also very tedious.

I have observed an interesting way that colors appear in the causal aura, which I call the *isle* or *island.* If we look at one of these islands in three dimensions, it will appear to be a dense-colored band around the person at a certain level of the body but with a different color completely surrounding that band. In cross section, or in two-dimensional representation, this island will look like a cable, with the center one color and the insulation another color. Over the years, I have come to get a feeling for the meaning of these islands. They seem to represent events in the past in which this soul was held back from expressing something.

A person once came to me for counseling, and I saw in his causal aura a purple area with red around it. I said to the person, "You cannot deal with any organized religion, can you?"

"Oh, no," he replied, "I have tried everything, but I cannot handle any organized religion."

"Also," I went on, "you cannot really deal with anything else that is organized. You are always rebelling against anything that imposes authority beyond your own authority." And the person had to admit that what I said was true. I explained my observations on the basis of what I had seen in the causal aura: "It seems that there was a stage of your life where you were forced by vital force, by physical force, to integrate, whatever and whenever that might have been." The red edge around the purple meant that there was force applied.

On another occasion, I was counseling a man to whom I said, "You must have problems with money. You can't hold onto money."

He said, "Yes, you're right. One hand gets money, and it's already spent by the other. It never warms my right hand because it's already been handed out by my left. I hate money. I don't want to have anything to do with it. But how did you know?"

I said, "You have a brown island in your causal aura, with red around it. Metaphorically, I might say you must have been a tax collector in your former life. In this life, you don't want anything to do with money because you were forced to deal with it in the past."

If we saw a yellow island with a green band around it, the green band would represent growth, evolution, preservation. For the sake of preservation, that person was totally involved in the rational.

That is how I use the causal aura in counseling. There is very little more I can tell you about it. However, we must be careful when we talk about former existences because past lives are certainly not the only explanation for some of the knowledge that people have of events from the past.

One investigation concerned a four-year-old Turkish boy who claimed that he had been murdered. He went several hundred miles away from where he was living and pointed out a barn where he claimed the body was buried. The investigators found the body there. The boy pointed out the person he claimed murdered him. In his former life, he had been the father of four adult sons; and as soon as he returned to the family's farm, he began to rule and regulate the entire household, including his claimed former wife. As a boy of four or five years old, he ruled the household like the adult of fifty-two who had been murdered!

In our investigations of past life experiences we have very rarely seen a person who has come back within a span of less than 700 or 800 years. Therefore, I suggest we be very cautious about life-readers who report ten lives for a subject in two or three centuries. The only instances in which people seem to come back sooner than 700 or 800 years is when they have been the victims of violent death—accidental death, murder, or suicide.

For two years, I was myself involved as a subject under regression. Every Sunday morning from nine o'clock to one o'clock, I was under deep hypnosis. We could not find any life experiences between this present one and one that was in 550 B.C. I was a gypsy, a Berber, and I spoke Arabic during the hypnotic sessions. The researchers could not understand me; they did not even know what language I was speaking. Finally, they borrowed some Arabic dictionaries and started reading words out to me. I did not understand what they were saying, but I was correcting their pronunciation. At last they brought in Ahmed el Senussi, a psychologist who lives in Ojai, California, to speak Arabic to me, and I answered him. Three weeks before he was brought in, I had stated that I was a Berber, that it was 550 B.C., and that I lived in a certain area in the mountains. When he came to talk to me, he said he could not understand what I was saying because I was speaking in a Berber dialect that had not been spoken since 300 B.C. That was quite a confirmation!

However, this does not necessarily prove a former life. It may be possible to resonate with occurrences out of the past, to be in tune psychically with someone else's life as if it were your own. So, we must be very careful not to jump to conclusions about past lives on the basis of such evidence.

## The Cosmic (Spiritual) Auras

The *cosmic* and *spiritual auras* (the actual names are interchangeable) are very difficult to see. I can say very little about them because I have not yet learned very much about what they mean, although I am sure eventually we may be able to observe more about them.

However, I have observed cases in which these auras have a definite meaning. Over the last several years, I have seen more and more people who have a very bright cosmic field; these people have been younger people, the so-called flower children of the coming Age of Aquarius.

When I have been able to distinguish the base colors of the cosmic field in these young people, something distinctive has made them stand out. What I have seen in that base color that sets them apart is very fine gold sparkles, like gold dust, giving the field a slight iridescence. The base color might be a very subtle—fine green or very subtle purple or blue —but they all have these same golden sparkles. It is as if you were in a dark room and the sun was shining through a slit in the curtain; a ray of light comes streaming into the dark room, and you see all the dust particles floating in it, and in their motion these dust particles twinkle like little golden speckles. That is what I have seen in these people's cosmic or spiritual auras.

I began to notice that there was something in common among all these people. These golden-speckled cosmic fields are found only in the younger generation, and all the people who have them seem to have similar feelings. In counseling sessions, they express the feeling that they do not belong on this planet Earth, that they do not know what they are supposed to be doing here. They seem to be wondering what they are doing here; it is as if they are all strangers in a strange land. I suggest that these people are souls incarnated from perhaps some other planet or cosmos of a high spiritual quality but who have difficulty adapting to the values of this planet. My youngest child, who is now nine years old (born May 13, 1970), is one of these Aquarian children with a gold-speckled aura. She is very headstrong and already seems to be setting herself up as my teacher, with an all-wise knowingness that seems beyond even the uncanny wisdom characteristic of children. When my wife was pregnant, I could see this gold-speckled aura emanating from her belly, and I knew the child would be one of these cosmic souls.

Figure 5 shows the arrangement of the seven auric fields. Always bear in mind that the actual human aura exists in three dimensions.

## Auric Diagnosis

Before I proceed with a discussion of how the aura can be used in diagnosing illness, let me emphasize something that I already have said and that I will repeat throughout this book: *It is very important to understand that before you can see anyone else's energy field, you will have to look through your own,* so your own had better be very, very subtle or transparent.

For example, let us assume that someone wakes me up at 6:30 A.M., just a half hour after I have gone to bed (I need very little sleep and

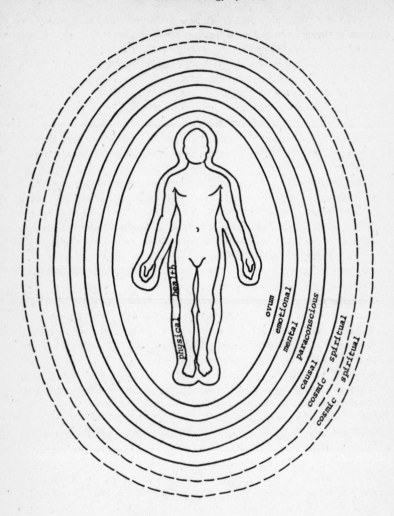

**FIGURE 5: THE SEVEN AURIC FIELDS**

often do not go to bed until nearly dawn), asking me to tell him what is in his energy field. I might say to him, "My! You certainly have a dark energy field around you!" What I'm actually seeing, of course, is the result of my own energy field, which is dark and murky; I have not even pulled the curtains up yet, and the fog has not lifted from my consciousness.

If we are going to use the aura as a diagnostic tool, we must always have our own energy fields under perfect observation, and we must never make a statement about anyone else's aura unless our own is so bright and transparent that it is like clear glass. If you are sick or tired, that is not the time to observe anyone else's energy field.

It has always amazed me to see people whose bodies are sick and deformed from the careless way they live, from improper diet and lack of discipline, who say to other people, "This is wrong with you, and that's wrong with you." I know they have to look through their own energy fields first, and quite often I wonder if they are not telling the other person some of the things they are seeing in their own auras. So, I caution you to be very careful, to be very sure that you are aware of your own energy field before you try to interpret what you see in that of another person.

Thus far, we have discussed each of the layers of the aura as a separate indication of what is going on in an individual's physical, emotional, mental, or spiritual state. In reality, of course, all the layers of the aura are interrelated. Let us say there is a brownish, murky bronze color around the heart in the emotional aura; there is still some golden orange showing through, but the color is largely dark and muddy. This means that there is some disease in the heart area. Of course, this heart disease will show up on the physical level as well. The physical aura, as you know, has no colors in it; but around the region of the heart and the thymus gland, you will observe dark spots in the physical aura. When we see a dark, muddy color in the heart region in the emotional aura, we know we have to look at the physical heart and thymus gland as well. On the other hand, you might discover the disorder first in the physical aura, and you will then note that the emotional aura is also darker in the same area. There is a correlation in every physiological condition. It is impossible to have a beautiful, glowing, subtle emotional aura when you have a terribly sick body. We therefore have several cross-references when we observe the aura. The only part of the aura that has no cross-references is the paraconscious aura, taken by itself, because the paraconscious aura represents the person's condition in his/her unconscious state. If, however, the mental aura shows a single blended color, with some merging with the paraconscious aura, then we know that the person has brought some of the aspects of his/her paraconscious through the mental into the emotional and that the emotional similarly will affect the physiological state. The reverse is, of course, also possible; the physiological state of a person may get better, and the emotional aura will get clearer, which will make it easier to work with a blended mind, and there will be a blending of the colors in the mental aura.

I have seen some individuals whose emotional auras are mirror images of their paraconscious auras. Such an aura marks a very high type of person. There are many saints walking among us, in all stations of life, from garbagemen to physicians to holy men. But these saints have healthy bodies. We have all heard stories about people who have become spiritual leaders and who have allowed their bodies to take on the karma of other people and who have died of some disease such as cancer. This makes no sense. I cannot take your karma upon my own shoulders; you cannot escape your karma, no matter what, because only you can do your own lessons. If I do your homework for you, you will not have learned anything from it. The only way you can graduate is by doing your own homework, to graduate from your own ignorance. Therefore, people who proclaim that they take on others' karmas for the love of them, do not really love their fellow humans deeply enough.

Let us take a detailed look at a hypothetical case in which the aura is used in diagnosis. A variety of colors can be seen in the emotional aura. Remember that these colors actually form three-dimensional bands around the physical body; they are not two-dimensional as in the drawing. What can we tell about this person on the basis of the colors in the emotional aura?

In the area of the root chakra is the color blue, which is the color of the throat chakra and represents expressive energy or will power. In this case, will power is being used, not to express energy, but to hold it back, to repress it. When the blue moves down, going below the throat chakra, you know will power is being pushed down, and suppression is taking place. In this person, the will power is being used to suppress the sexual energy of the root chakra.

Around the solar plexus area we see the color pink. Pink is the color of love, of reserve energy. A lot of extra emotional energy is being pumped into the solar plexus area, and so the person is in a highly emotional state; but these emotions have not penetrated farther up and undergone transmutation at the heart chakra, where they would be turned into subtler energies. Such heightened emotionality in the solar plexus area, as you know, can lead to physical problems such as indigestion and ulcers.

Purple, the color of integration, or spirituality, is at the area of the throat chakra. It is at this chakra that energies are expressed through volition. This is the sort of person who will act as if everything has to be spiritual but who misunderstands the meaning of spirituality. He/-she is bringing the purple from the crown chakra down to the throat chakra, where he/she is trying to bring it out. So, this person is trying to express the spiritual, but he/she is not really living it.

This person also has pure yellow above his/her head. (For the sake of simplicity, we have eliminated the ray in this drawing, so the yellow is in the emotional aura, rather than representing the ray.) I have found that when a person is in beta a lot of the time, there is a kind of yellowish glow around the brain; when he/she is in alpha, there is a bluish glow around the brain; in theta, there is a purplish glow; and in delta, the emanation becomes a whitish gray or silver gray. Even the Menninger Foundation has confirmed that they see blue around the brain when a person is in alpha, although they have not been able to confirm the other colors for me.

The person in the drawing has pure yellow above his/her head, so he/she is in beta a great deal of the time. His/her crown chakra is radiating purple, but only at the throat area where he/she is trying to express it. The yellow, which is associated with consciousness, with the heart chakra, he/she is trying to bring up toward the pineal gland; so he/she has his/her heart on top of his/her pineal gland, on top of his/her head! His/her consciousness is all located at the top of the head, which indicates a lot of cerebral action.

Between the yellow at the top of the head and the purple in the throat area, we see green in the area of the pituitary, or the brow chakra. Green is the color of the solar plexus and carries the idea, "I want to grow." But how is this person growing? He/she is not giving out his/her life-preserving energies but is keeping them all to him/herself. He/she is like a rose in a garden, surrounded by thousands of other roses, who says, "I want to grow; I want all the food." This person is a narcissist. He/she holds everything in and wants to grow only spiritually. Somehow he/she has got the idea that his/her body does not need to be involved in this growth. He/she has the emotions from the solar plexus growth state all bound up with his/her concern about spiritual growth; he/she is probably one of those starry-eyed people who does not feel he/she needs to be involved from below, to release his/her energies. He/she is very unrealistic.

A person with such colors in the emotional aura would be expected to be physically in a tight, rigid state. His/her problems will show up not only in the emotional aura but also in the physical aura. As you can see in the chart on the cover, there are dark spots around all the joints in the physical aura. This person has arthritis, a stiffness and rigidity in the joints. He/she also has stomach problems. His/her energy is so clotted up that he/she has a dark band around the waist in the solar plexus area in the physical aura. He/she will probably have problems with constipation as well and will undoubtedly have sexual problems; if the person is male, he may have prostate troubles, for example. All of his/her sexual energy is being kept down and cannot move up in a healthy expression of energy flow.

Furthermore, because of the emotional and mental state this individual is in, he/she is constantly in the beta brain wave and is susceptible to migraines. The energies are all held in the cerebral area. As we noted in Chapter 1, such excessive cerebral activity also draws the blood to the brain, resulting in bad circulation to the rest of the body.

What might we see in the mental aura of our hypothetical patient? This person operates intellectually and does not allow his/her intuition to come out at all; he/she holds it in. In such a case, the inner part of the mental aura will be deep, dark orange, and the outer part will be very bright yellow. If the person improves after treatment, the colors will blend and the mental aura would be a beautiful golden yellow. (If the colors are reversed, this will be a totally intuitive person who is not able to use the rational mind to put his/her intuitions into expression, to make them a reality.)

Thus, at one glance, auric vision permits us to observe an individual's mental, emotional, and physical states. Of course, you would not want to restrict yourself to observing the physical, emotional, and mental auras; you would go on to the subtlest auras as well.

What would the therapist do when confronted by the subject on the cover? The only way to communicate with such a person is by some other than verbal means. You cannot talk with such persons; they have their own opinions and are not interested in hearing yours. So, the first thing you would do in a therapy session is bombard him/her with bright white light. This not only protects him/her from you but also protects you from him/her. When I stand in front of a class, I do not want the students' problems to disturb me. I bombard the class with bright white light, which means that I first have to activate it and get it moving and get it out so that it is very beneficial for me. At the same time, I become nonattached, and whatever is happening happens in the white light, and I cannot be affected by it in a negative way. I expand myself throughout the room with all that energy so that the class will feel me, so that my beingness will affect everyone in the room. Anyone who deals with health must radiate his/her health out him/herself. So, if a person comes to you for help, you first must bombard that person with light and bombard the room you are working in with light. It is as if you have to be in a state of excitation all the time.

When I am traveling and arrive in a new hotel room, I do not want to be involved in what went on there before me, so I whitewash the room by shining white light into it. Wherever I go, I am constantly whitewashing; and if that does not work fast enough, I will also chant the om. Sound has the same effect; it breaks down all the densities of energy around you.

You can tell in therapy when you are having an effect on a person. You have embraced the person with the white light, which starts to regenerate his/her systems. No verbalization is needed to accomplish this. If the person's aura does not get lighter in color, then your energy is not working; it is not high enough to regenerate that person. Maybe you do not have enough energy available at that moment to help regenerate that person.

## Dating Events from the Aura

Through many years of observation, I have discovered another interesting source of information in the human energy field: what I call the *growth pattern* in the aura. From below the sacral area, down into the ground where you cannot see the aura anymore, the emotional aura is a brownish green color, usually somewhat lighter toward the outside. It is in this part of the emotional aura that we can observe the growth pattern. We can see vortices, which are also slightly visible in the physical aura, including the ovum. Through experience, I have learned that these vortices of energy surrounding a person are like growth rings in trees and that each ring represents a year in time. Let us say that suddenly, four years ago, our subject had a spiritual rebirth, a tremendous transition in his/her life. In the growth area, the aura would begin, from that point on, to look a lighter green. It might be kelly green to start, and where the rebirth occurred, it would suddenly get subtler, more of a chartreuse color, and you can start to count lines in it because every line becomes a subtler color. It is therefore possible to determine the approximate date at which important events took place or when a disease started by counting back on these growth rings. If the change took place four and a half years ago, the color change will be seen four and a half lines in from the outer part of the emotional aura.

## The Flow of Energies and Auric Color Theory

In Chapter 1, we saw that light is a form of nourishment for the human organism and that as it moves down through the chakras, it is broken down into different qualities that nourish the different systems of the body. Below the heart, the light becomes progressively denser and more material. It then goes through a process of activation in the generative system, at the root chakra. Practically all diseases have their foundation in this basement area, where energies have taken on their densest form and not enough filtering may take place in this density. I often call this area, where energy exchange tends to get bogged down, the *molasses*. As it moves up, it becomes more fluid; and past the heart chakra, it becomes light. The process, then, is from light to fire to substance or from substance to fire to light. If you bring the light down —for example, if you bring the purple from the crown chakra down to the solar plexus—it will look darker and more dense in the emotional aura. Dark, muddy colors show the influence of higher colors that actually cannot function lower down. So, we really need to bring the lower ones up to make them lighter, not the higher ones down to make them denser. The normal process is a flow in and through and out, and anything that tries to make a bypass—from the crown center to the solar plexus, for example, forgetting about the throat and the heart— will produce a stagnation and will impede the healthy flow of energies. The energies have to go through the heart, and after they have gone down through the heart, they become denser.

We have seen in the emotional aura that when the colors of the higher chakras have been brought down, that means you are repressing the energies. Taking an example of the opposite case, what would it mean if a person brings the pink up around the shoulders? Pink is the color of emotion; when we see a lot of pink in the emotional aura, we know we are dealing with a highly emotional individual. But now the pink is up around the shoulders, at the level of the throat chakra. The throat chakra is no longer blue; it is now pink. Such a person no longer has sympathy, but empathy; he/she has brought his/her emotions up through the heart chakra, the seat of consciousness, and is now expressing them. This is a desirable state of affairs.

The ideal situation is to have the chakras work upward in their expression in the emotional aura. It is a good sign, for example, for blue to be seen above the throat chakra; now the will power is directed to a higher order of things. In philosophical terms, we might label this state as being not "my will" anymore but "Thy will" that will be done. This is moving toward the transpersonal state. On the other hand, whenever the blue goes below the throat chakra, you know will power is being pushed down and suppression or repression is taking place.

Let us suppose that we see a very bright orange in the heart chakra. This indicates that the red orange has moved from the gonad area, through the pink of the spleen chakra and the green of the solar plexus, and it is now bombarding the heart chakra. Such a person is in flames. He/she has become transpersonal, meaning that he/she has gone beyond his/her own personality; he/she is "dis-identifying" with his/her own personality and is now identifying with his/her universal self, in other words, with his/her divine self, higher self, or God-self. However, this is not the highest state. When a person reaches Christ consciousness, which simply means a state of enlightenment, there is no fire anymore, there is only light. Then we see the pure white of saintliness, the halo.

How might such higher states of consciousness appear in the paraconscious aura? Let us say that we see pink in the solar plexus area in the paraconscious aura. Pink is the color of emotion, of love energy. When the pink has moved up to the solar plexus area, that means that the solar plexus is now under the influence of this energy; the aura only reflects what is actually happening in you, although in this case it may be largely unconscious. When the pink is in the solar plexus area, you feel what has been described as a "vexation of spirit," a longing, a craving to be with a higher power. The difference between a normal, physically based emotional state and a paraconscious emotional state is that the paraconscious state involves lower frequencies and higher amplitudes of energy. This is when we say we are in touch with the unattainable, when we are having a peak experience. In such a state, we might see a very bright gold in the heart area of the paraconscious aura and a beautiful pink in the solar plexus area. The emotional energy represented by the color pink is being used, not to express physically based drives, but rather to get in touch with a higher power, with what we might call *God* or *spirit*. This is still an emotional experience, still grounded in the physical body, but it is a condition of joy, a high peak experience.

## Preparing to See the Aura

In Chapter 4, I will describe some exercises that will improve your physical vision and therefore help you to see the human aura. You may still have some questions about how the aura really looks. You might think that because the various auras are in layers, one over the other, you would not be able to distinguish which layer is which. Actually, it is like looking through a very transparent jawbreaker candy, made up of different colors and flavors; even though you have an outer layer of color on the outside, it is so subtle that when you look farther into the next one, the density is different, and therefore you can distinguish one layer from another. The various layers of density will be particularly visible if you look at a person from the side.

It does become more difficult to distinguish the layers when they start to merge, when one layer becomes so highly charged that the next starts to blend with it, for example, when the emotional aura begins to blend with the mental, and then you also start to see a merging of the mental with the paraconscious. When you see this, you know the person is fulfilling his or her purpose, that what comes through intuitively is directing his/her mind and actions, and that his/her emotions are regulated by his/her unconscious-paraconscious mind. This is a good thing to see. What you would see in the physical aura in such a case is the aura becoming brighter and brighter, the corona becoming wider, and the ovum becoming much lighter and subtler until it becomes a cleaner, paler ivory than it was before. Even in such a case, you can look through the aura and distinguish the different layers once you learn to see them.

When you use meditation and exercises to raise your energy patterns so that your consciousness and your energy are expanding, you are automatically going to affect all the different layers of your aura. It all becomes brighter, until eventually the layers start blending. The ideal situation would be if there were only one layer, no longer divided into different densities or subtleties.

Of course, the closer you can come to having such a high level of energy, such a blending of your own aura, the more accurate your perceptions of the energy fields around other people will be. This is why it is important to be healthy—not only physically healthy but mentally, emotionally, and spiritually healthy—when we attempt to observe the auras of others.

# 4 : Eye Exercises for Auric Vision

## The Physiology of Expanded Vision

Human beings generally use only a small percentage of the light that enters the eye because of improper use of the eyes, laziness, and ignorance of the eye's function. It has been said that only 10 percent of the light that enters the eye is actually utilized.

When light enters the eye, it hits the retina, in which two different types of cells are found: The rods deal with light and dark perception; they are highly sensitive to the presence of light but cannot respond to color. The cones are concerned with color vision; there are three different types of cones, which respond respectively to yellow, blue, and red wavelengths. When light strikes the retina, its energy is absorbed by the rods and cones in the area it hits. There is a pigment in the rods (and presumably in the cones also) that, when light is absorbed by the rod, breaks down into simpler compounds. The pigment bleaches out during this breakdown, changing from purple to a yellowish color. Something in this chain of events triggers a release of electrical energy; the energy released in this manner by the rods and cones moves through the optic nerve. The optic nerve is different from any other nerve in the body; it is like a tunnel, actually made up of many individual nerve fibers. The energy carried by the optic nerve activates the brain and, according to the frequencies and amplitudes of the light that has entered the eye, starts a certain rhythm. The brain radiates out this rhythmic energy, which is now synthesized on the visual area of the cerebral cortex, which is your screen. As soon as this synthesized picture is reflected back, you say, "I see."

How can we increase the activity of the rods and cones? By activating the muscles of the eyelids and of the eye itself, we expose a greater number of rods and cones to the incoming light because the light will not be hitting just one focal point on the retina. The eye exercises described in this chapter are intended to teach you to use the muscles of your eyes, thereby stimulating more rods and cones. The more energy that gets from the eyes into the optic nerve, the more the brain will be activated; the screen can therefore synthesize more than it did before, and you will see more.

Physics tells us that the visible spectrum is from a wavelength of 400 nanometers to a wavelength of 700 nanometers. However, these limits represent an average; certainly, there are people with no particular gifts who can see higher or lower than this range. One of the things that limits our ability to see beyond the so-called visible spectrum is our mental acceptance that we cannot see beyond this range (see Figure 6). If we can let go of that preconception about the limitations of our visual ability, we should be able to expand the range of our vision.

Some time ago, I was involved in an experiment with Professor John Adams, a geophysicist at the University of Washington in Seattle who interprets the infrared pictures of the geological situation on earth that have been taken from satellites. In his laboratory, I participated in a visual experiment in which he sent out a ray of light and I told him

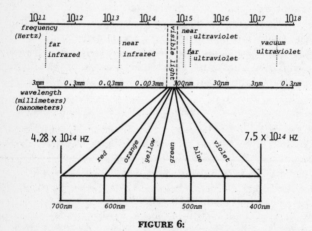

**FIGURE 6:**

**THE VISIBLE SPECTRUM AND NEIGHBORING FREQUENCIES**

From *Encyclopedia Americana*, 1973, vol. 25, p. 467.

when I started seeing it and what I saw. He recorded my observations on a computerized graph that was synchronized with the record of the frequencies of the light he sent out, and when we later looked at the graph, it showed that I had been able to see light from 335 nanometers, which is in the shortwave, or ultraviolet, range, 65 nanometers below the visible spectrum, up to 1,700 nanometers, which is in the infrared, 1,000 nanometers above the visible spectrum! Professor Adams also tried the experiment and was amazed to discover that although he could not see in the ultraviolet, he was able to get up to 1,335, well beyond the visible spectrum. To do this, he had to throw away a previous concept and keep an open mind; then he, too, was able to experience this expanded vision.

The eye exercises described in this chapter can expand your vision if you are able to keep an open mind about the possibilities. These are purely physiological, not metaphysical, exercises. There is a certain amount of discipline involved in learning to do the exercises correctly without trying too hard to see some results. The breathing exercises that should precede the eye exercises will similarly help to activate your system by providing plenty of oxygen. Taken altogether, these exercises should result in brighter color vision and increased perception. Even if you never see auras after doing these exercises, you should at least gain an improvement in your eyesight, provided that you work at it.

## General Instructions for the Eye Exercises

In dealing with the human aura, there are two notions we must overcome. First, you have probably been told that such things do not exist, so you will have to deal with your own limiting belief system. Second, you may have been told that even if the aura does exist, you will never be able to see it. The purpose of working with the eye charts described in this chapter is to improve your vision, to increase the muscular control and strength of the eyes and thereby stimulate the rods and cones to a greater degree. By strengthening your vision, the eye exercises can help you to see auras. Research may eventually confirm my own suspicion, based on my observations over more than thirty-five years, that whereas most people use only 15 or 20 percent of the available rods and cones in their eyes, people with auric vision use perhaps 35 percent or more of the available rods and cones.

The charts are simply a guide to help you learn to control your eyes. If you discover you can control your eyes in the ways suggested without the charts, so much the better; the charts are for those people who need some help to discover the eyes' abilities.

These exercises must be prefaced with a warning. *Do not imagine that you can use these methods lightly.* This work requires your sincere cooperation. If the purpose of doing these exercises is to make you capable of observing human energies, you must be sincere in your desire, first, for self-improvement and, second, for getting to know your fellow humans better and to interact with and help them. Observing human energies can be an especially valuable diagnostic and therapeutic tool for people who are involved in the health professions and in counseling.

These exercises should be done every day; otherwise, you will have no way of knowing if you are really improving. The charts should be used at home, whenever you are free of all distractions. Do the exercises in a very well lit room because you need reflection, but avoid any glare.

With all these exercises, the harder you try, the less you will experience. Results come from intense concentration without volition, a state of consciousness generally corresponding to the low alpha and theta frequencies.

Using the dimensions given, make your own charts out of construction paper. The charts should be hung on a wall that is free from distracting objects, with the center of each chart at eye level and about six feet away from you.

There are four charts; each has a different role in exciting your perception of colors. I have also included a breathing exercise, the lion's breath, that should precede each eye exercise, as well as two finger exercises to supplement the benefits to your eye muscles. Charts 1, 2, and 4 are all black and white. You might think that in order to see colors, the charts should have colors in them. But black has absorbed all the colors in light, and white reflects all the light. So, in black and white, all the colors are there; it is up to you to discover them and take them out of their black or white state.

If you wear glasses, you should do the zooming exercises and the other exercises with your glasses on. If you wear contact lenses, you should remove them during the eye exercises, as well as during the lion's breath. When you become capable of doing the exercises readily and have some feeling that you are perceiving more clearly, remove your glasses, and see if you can achieve the same results without them, perhaps with a little extra effort. These exercises can improve your vision in general, as well as enable you to see auras.

Once you have become familiar with the kinds of muscular and visual activities that are stimulated by the charts, you can use a tree or a point on the wall or something on the horizon, and do the same things with them that you do with the charts. However, the charts give you a point of concentration and discipline by teaching you to stay within the limits of the design on the chart.

When you work with these charts every day, you will begin to see faint, fuzzy colors, which you may immediately discount as being the result of muscle strain or afterimages. Yet, the colors you are looking for will at first come in precisely this manner. One way to distinguish afterimages is that they will always float in front of the chart. If you see colors in the same plane as the chart, pay passive attention. After some progress, you may go through a stage where you will see rainbows everywhere. Because of the intent gazing involved in these exercises, you may see images or colors from the charts superimposed on the wall or on empty space, when you suddenly look away from the chart. This stage will pass. These are afterimages of what you saw in the charts and may be your first indication that you are beginning to get some results.

As you go through the exercises, make smaller copies of the charts on white paper. As you begin to see colors, use crayons or colored pencils to duplicate on these charts what you have observed in doing the exercises. This is very important because if and when your new visual experiences start occurring, you may doubt whether you are observing something different from what you used to see. By marking down your color experiences on copies of the charts as they occur to you, you will have a record of your progress. This feedback will help you to gain confidence in your organism and its powers.

In the instructions that follow, I first give the exercises to be done with each of the charts, but I do not say what you are likely to observe. In this way, I avoid giving you any presuggestions. In a separate section, "Feedback from Eye Charts," you will find descriptions of the color experiences you are likely to have. Work with the charts to observe colors in them for yourself before you read the descriptions in the feedback section.

*Under no circumstances should you do these exercises longer than ten or fifteen minutes at a time.* Take a rest for about twenty minutes at the end of an exercise period. Eye fatigue will tell you when to stop because you are exercising the muscles of your eyes more vigorously than you are accustomed to doing. Ideally, the exercises should not need to be done more than twice a day, in the morning and at night, for example. The charts should be used in the order given, with sufficient rest after each. I would not recommend that you go on to the later exercises until you have seen at least some colors with Chart 1. However, if you have repeatedly tried Chart 1 and then 2 for ten or fifteen minutes each with very little result, then go on to Chart 3, which is the easiest to get results with. Then, when you go back to the earlier charts, you may see something there, and that will encourage you.

### Breathing Exercise: Lion's Breath

Before doing the eye exercises with the charts, it is always recommended that you do the breathing exercises taught in *Voluntary Controls*, namely, paradoxical breathing or, if you are not able to sustain paradoxical breathing, diaphragmatic breathing. It is very important to do these breathing exercises because the activation of your system, including your eyes, depends on the proper fuel, oxygen.

After doing the general breathing exercises, you should next do a special breathing exercise derived from yoga, known as the *lion's breath*. This exercise is specifically designed to force oxygen into the head and behind the eyes. When you first try the lion's breath, you might want to check for an improvement in your vision by looking at a colored object in your surroundings before you begin and then looking at it after doing the breathing exercise. Immediately after doing the lion's breath, you will find that the eyes have become relaxed and everything looks brighter. As with the eye exercises themselves, even if this breathing exercise does not lead ultimately to your being able to see auras, it can at least produce an improvement in your eyesight if you practice it regularly.

The lion's breath should be done in a sitting position because it may affect your equilibrium. Slowly take a deep breath, using your abdomen to suck in the air, and then bring the air up, as if to exhale, but instead put a throat lock on the breath, and gag. In the beginning, you will probably make some sound effects as you gag, so you may want to do this in privacy. After you become accustomed to the exercise, you will learn that it is not necessary to make a gagging noise.

In the classical yoga posture, the tongue is thrust backward to heighten the gag effect. For this exercise, you do not need to go that far. Instead of thrusting the tongue backward, you stick it out. The more you gag, the more your tongue will stick out. Again, hold your breath; act as if you are going to exhale, but hold it back, and force it up into the skull cavities instead.

You can practice this exercise at other times during the day, for example, whenever you go to the bathroom. It will help your bowel movements and improve your circulation. So, go ahead and gag a little!

If you wear glasses, you can keep them on during this exercise as long as they do not pop off your nose. If you wear contact lenses, take them out, although you may need to replace them for the later eye exercises, at least at first, until you can do without them.

*Description.* You can make this chart out of construction paper. Start with a 15-inch black square. In the middle of this, put a 9-inch white square. Finally, in the middle of the white square put a 3-inch black square. Place this chart, with the center at eye level, about six feet away, on an uncluttered wall in a well-lit room.

*Breathing Exercise.* Start by doing the lion's breath to send oxygen to the brain and eyes.

*Step 1: Concentration and Decentration.* Imagine a little white dot at the very center of the chart. Focus your eyes on this imaginary center spot. When you are properly concentrated, you will be completely absorbed in the whole chart and decentrated from everything around it. (At least at first, it will help if there are no distracting objects on the wall adjacent to the chart.)

*Step 2: Zooming.* In order to learn to zoom in and zoom out on the chart, mentally bring the chart toward you, as if it were in motion, coming toward you and past you. When this is done properly, the chart will seem to become three-dimensional; the squares will become cubes, and it will appear that you are looking through the interior of a bellows that is moving past you as it expands. Then push the chart away from you mentally, so that the bellows appears to close and move away. This zoom effect is accomplished by using the muscles inside your eyes.

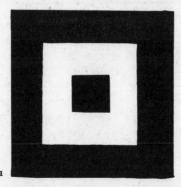

**FIGURE 7: CHART 1**

When you are zooming in and zooming out on the chart, you will feel the effects on the muscles in your eyes.

*Step 3: Vertical Sweep.* After you have established good zooming contact with the chart, focus on the center of the chart with both eyes. Raise both your eyes with a broad sweep to the top of the chart. Imagine that the chart is the wall of a room and that you are looking up to the angle it makes with the ceiling. You must see *all* the chart, and nothing but the chart, without focusing on any one part, and covering the whole area in a broad sweep. Next, sweep down to the bottom edge. Sweep your eyes up and down the chart. Imagine that your eyes are brooms and that you are sweeping the chart with equal force with each eye. Stay within the boundary of the black outer square.

In the beginning, you will need to practice this sweeping motion very slowly. If one eye is stronger than the other, you might want to practice with the weaker eye alone, to strengthen it. First, zoom in and zoom out. Then, close one eye, and scan in a broad sweep with one eye, then the other, working at each of them until both achieve the same speed. Once you have gotten a good speed going with each eye, do the exercise with both eyes.

*Step 4: Horizontal Sweep.* Do exactly the same sweeping motion, but now let both eyes sweep horizontally, once again making sure to take in all the chart. Go from the left edge to the right edge and back. You will notice that there is a difference in this pattern. When you move your eyes to the side, the outside eye will reach the edge first, and the other eye will stop in the middle. Try to accept the feeling of being divided in half; do not let one eye lead or dominate. This is not easy, but it is a preparation for the next step.

*Step 5: Combined Sweep.* Combine the vertical and horizontal motion by starting at the bottom of the chart, going up to the center, then out to the left edge, then across to the right edge, then back to the center, up to the top, and back to the bottom (see Figure 8). Although it sounds complicated, the pattern is actually quite easy. You can vary this combined motion, for example, starting at the top. In the beginning, this will go very slowly; you will have to become comfortable with the early parts of the exercise (up and down, left and right) before you can get up a good speed on the combined sweep.

The goal of this exercise is to learn to do it quickly because the more speed you achieve, the more you will start observing things that are not at first apparent in the chart. Speed will stimulate and excite the eyes.

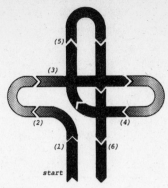

**FIGURE 8: COMBINED SWEEP**

At first, you will need a couple of ten- or fifteen-minute sessions on each separate movement before you can do them quickly and thoroughly enough to put them together into the combined sweep. Be sure to rest adequately after these ten- or fifteen-minute practice periods. Do not be impatient with yourself; you have used your eyes in this fashion very little (if at all) in your life.

Once you can do the combined sweep fast enough and with proper concentration, you will begin to see colors. Record what you see on a copy of the chart.

Discipline is important in this exercise. The more you look for color, the less you will see because you put your thinking process in the way of pure response to stimulation. Even if you think you have seen no colors, you may perceive afterimages of colors after you stop looking at the chart. This is the test of achievement in the exercises. The afterimage is a reaction to what you were stimulated to see; if you did not see anything, there would be no afterimage.

Another test is to look away from the chart and then look right back. If the rods and cones of your eyes were truly stimulated intensely, you may be able to see the colors briefly.

The feedback section will show what color patterns you may experience when you work with the chart, but do not refer to that section until you have had the chance to observe some results for yourself.

Some people will not get any results from this exercise at first. They need some more immediate feedback to see what is happening in their heads and their eyes when they are zooming. If you feel you are not getting any results from Chart 1, do part 1 of the finger exercise (page 79).

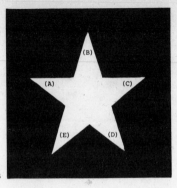

**FIGURE 9: CHART 2**

*Description.* This chart consists of a white five-pointed star on a 15-inch black square. From one point of the star to its opposite point, along a straight line, is 11 inches. The distance between adjacent points is about 6 3/4 inches. Hang the chart six feet away with its center at eye level.

*Breathing Exercise.* Do the lion's breath.

*Step 1: Zooming.* Zoom in and out on the chart a couple of times until you have some familiarity with it. Keep the whole chart in focus all the time.

*Step 2: Gaze and Float (8–4 Count).* Start at point A (see Figure 9). Concentrate and decentrate on the point. Imagine that the point is the center of a circle about two inches in diameter, and gaze at it for 8 counts (each count is equal to about one second). In the black space between A and B, imagine four equally spaced points. Counting 1, 2, 3, 4, look at each imaginary point, as you float from A to B. Then look at B for 8 counts, again imagining a two-inch circle with point B as its center. Repeat the process, floating from point to point on 4 counts, until you return to A. Then go immediately to point C, gaze for 8 counts, and repeat the whole process, but this time going around the star in a counterclockwise direction. Rest for 15 to 20 counts.

*Step 3: Gaze and Float (4–2 Count).* Repeat Step 2 completely, but this time use 4 counts on the points of the star and 2 counts in between. Rest.

*Step 4: Gaze and Float (2–1 Count).* Repeat the same process, but use 2 counts on the points of the star and 1 in between. Rest.

After each stage of gazing and floating, rest for 15 to 20 counts. After doing all four steps, rest at least half an hour.

Once you begin observing things when you do this exercise, record the results on a copy of the chart. The feedback section describes what you should experience, but again, do not look at this section until you have gotten some results for yourself.

*Description.* This chart consists of a 5-inch-diameter circle of royal blue or dark powder blue on a 15-inch white square. Hang it six feet away with the center at eye level.

*Breathing Exercise.* Do the lion's breath.

*Step 1: Zooming.* Gaze at the center of the blue circle. Zoom in and out. Once you have established good zooming contact with the chart, you may start seeing some things.

*Step 2: Clockwise Circle.* Move the eyes around the edge of the blue circle faster and faster. Try to follow the outer edge of the blue circle against the white background. In the beginning, you might move your head slightly so that you become aware of the feeling of the motion. Then, do it just with your eyes. This will be rather slow at first. Rest your eyes for a couple of seconds, and repeat this part of the exercise, first focusing and zooming in and out, then moving around the circle clockwise. Before you try the next motion (which is counterclockwise), you will want to develop good clockwise speed. A good speed is ten times around the circle in one minute.

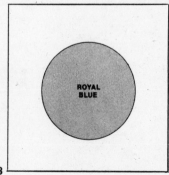

**FIGURE 10: CHART 3**

*Step 3: Counterclockwise Circle.* Repeat the circular motion, following the edge of the blue circle in a counterclockwise direction. Get the feeling of moving your eyes, rather than your head. You must feel that your eyes are doing the rolling, although in the beginning you may feel some strain in your eye muscles. Keep working for increased speed, moving in both clockwise and counterclockwise directions, with adequate rest periods in between.

After working with this chart, close your eyes, and look at the afterimages. Sometimes the colors around the circle will also appear as afterimages first, but they will be in the opposing colors.

As with all the charts, do not do this exercise for more than ten or fifteen minutes at a time. Then rest at least twenty minutes.

Record your results on a copy of the chart. What you may experience is described in the feedback section.

*Description.* This chart, like the first two, is black and white, with no colors. It consists of a black rectangle on the left, 15 inches high by 9 inches wide, side by side with a white rectangle of the same dimensions on the right. Inside the black rectangle is a white oval, and inside the white rectangle is a white oval outlined in black. Inside the oval on the white side (but not the one on the black side) is a black horizontal lens or eye-shaped form (see Figure 11). Hang this chart six feet away, with its center at eye level.

*Breathing Exercise.* Do the lion's breath.

*Step 1: Zoom and Sweep, One Side and Both Sides, One Eye.* Cover one eye. Focus the other eye on the left half of the chart. Make the white

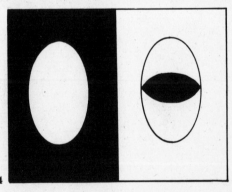

**FIGURE 11: CHART 4**

oval zoom in and zoom out. Sweep that eye up and down on the left half of the chart. Then have it sweep both sides together, up and down.

*Step 2: Zoom and Sweep, One Side and Both Sides, Other Eye.* Repeat the same steps with the other eye alone.

*Step 3: Sweep, Whole Chart, Both Eyes.* With both eyes, sweep the whole chart up and down. Avoid having one eye stay on one side of the chart. Work to increase your speed as you sweep faster and faster, up and down.

You may get the feeling of being cross-eyed after doing this exercise, because it is not easy. I advise doing it first with each eye separately to see which eye is more perceptive and more capable of doing it; then do it with both eyes when you feel they are both perceiving equally.

If you do the exercise and do not get any results, keep gazing at the chart passively for a few minutes; you are likely to get the feedback then. You need to be patient. Remember, your eyes are getting very tired from doing something they are not accustomed to.

Record your observations on a copy of the chart. The colors you should perceive are discussed in the feedback section.

## Finger Exercise

First do the lion's breath.

*Part 1.* For people who need early feedback from zooming exercises, try this finger exercise.

Hold one index finger a couple of inches away from your eyes, and gaze at it. Then put your other index finger in front of the first. Now, without paying any attention to the first, closer finger, start moving the other finger away from you very slowly, following it with your eyes. Move this finger until it is at arm's length; then bring it back very slowly until it meets the first finger.

You may see some strange phenomena during this finger exercise, perhaps a transparent finger or two or three fingers. Do not pay attention to these. After doing this exercise, you should be able to close your eyes, imagine your finger to be in front of you, and reproduce in your mind's eye the experience of zooming in and out with the finger. When you open your eyes and try zooming with the chart, you should not have such difficulty.

*Part 2*. This part of the exercise, besides activating your rods and cones by increasing your eye movements, will also improve your peripheral vision.

Extend the index finger of your right hand, with the thumb tucked inside the palm. Place the index finger against your nose so the knuckle touches your nostril. Then do the same thing on the other side of your nose with the left hand. Gaze at the right index finger; this may make you feel slightly cross-eyed. Now, very slowly, move the other finger straight away from you, and look at this finger which is moving away. Still very slowly, bring the finger back, but instead of stopping, let it go past your eyes, and follow it without turning your head. Keep following the finger as you move it around and behind your head; it is as if you are looking through your head. Now bring the finger very slowly back to your nose.

After you have done this a couple of times, switch hands and do the exercise with the opposite finger.

The reason you focus on the first finger is to get your eyes to converge. When you start to look at the finger that moves, you will lose sight of the stationary finger. Also, when you start to focus on the finger that moves away, it may extend itself visually so that two fingers are coming at you, like a transparent image. You may see an energy field around your finger, which is its physical aura. As you continue to gaze at the finger, you may see a streak of light moving with it, as though you are seeing an energy field moving along with it.

After a period of intense focusing, the moving finger may become a phantom finger entirely, only the fingernail and the tip of the finger being visible; or your whole finger may disappear when you bring it back.

Of course, these results depend on the condition of your eyesight. Along with the results described, everything will look brighter after you do the exercise.


### Feedback from Eye Charts

*Chart 1*. The colors and spectra you see in the horizontal sweep should be the same in the vertical sweep but arranged differently, of course. In the vertical sweep (step 3), the colors will appear as vertical rainbows in the white area to each side of the black center square. In the horizontal sweep (step 4), the rainbows will be horizontal, in the white above, and below the center black square. In the combined sweep (step 5), you will see interlacing rainbows, a checkerboard of colors, throughout the entire white section, and eventually you will see a circle of colors like a color wheel.

*Chart 2.* On the 8–4 count, you will probably not see anything but gray. On the 4–2 count, the imaginary circles around each point take on a goldish white. When you move from point to point, you see a reddish pink glow in between. On the 2–1 count, you begin to get the feeling that the star has changed into a circle; later, you see all the colors of the spectrum in the circle. In the center of the white star, the lighter colors —light green, light pink, light blue, yellow—will appear. On the outer part of the star, the darker colors—deep purple, blue, green—appear. As you speed up the count, you will see gray, gold, and silver at the points, and as you further increase the tempo around the star, you may occasionally see golden flashes or sparks.

In the white area in the middle of the chart, some people see the image of an individual: a man, a woman, or a baby. Such images are coming from the unconscious. The exercise has stimulated the unconscious mind through activation of the visual cortex, which begins to release some intuitive images that have nothing to do with this particular exercise. The mental image is simply being reflected on the visual cortex. To counter such distractions, make an intensive effort at focusing first, before you start to do the exercise itself, in order to keep your eyes from playing optical games with you.

*Chart 3.* First, you will notice a golden sunburst all around the blue circle. Second, the ball becomes three-dimensional; you feel almost as if you can see behind it. Third, the faster you move your eyes, the more they seem to stand still. As you go faster and faster, eventually you will see colors arranged around the ball in eight equally spaced segments. At the top is red; then, going counterclockwise, the red turns into violet, then a white spot with changing colors, then blue, then green at the bottom, then yellow, then another white spot with changing colors on the left, then orange. As you become even more proficient with this chart, the white background will look lavender purplish, and the blue circle will look white.

With faster motion around the circle, the spectrum will rotate according to the speed of eye movement, as if there were three or four circles superimposed on each other, each of them having different colors that move in their places. However, the colors will remain in the same sequence in relation to each other as before.

This is the easiest of the four eye charts because the results come faster than with the square or the star. With those two charts, you get many afterimages; there are afterimages with the circle, too, but you can recognize them for what they are.

*Chart 4.* On the left side, you will see a green eye in the same place and with the same shape as the black eye in the middle of the right oval. Within the left oval, you will see concentric oval-shaped rings of color next to the black background, beginning with the darker colors on the outside: purple, indigo, blue, green. As you get toward the center of the white oval, the colors are lighter: yellow, orange, red. On the right side of the chart, the colors are reversed; the purple is on the inside, and the red is on the outside. On the right side you will also see, within the oval, a crescent-shaped spectrum of color above and below the eye, with the purple closest to the black of the eye and the red toward the outside.

## Observing the Aura

What results can you expect from doing the eye exercises? The charts are, after all, inanimate objects, and so there is not much variety to be had in observing them. Later on, when you begin viewing the energy fields around people, it will be an entirely different matter because there is such a great variety of changes taking place in human energy fields that it may be difficult to pick out even a general pattern in an individual.

One of my students, working with the charts for about twenty minutes a day, found that at the end of five weeks of practice, he was able to see a few distinct colors around a subject; I was able to confirm those colors as part of the subject's aura. Training to see the aura is not a simple task. Besides having the proper motivation and following the discipline of meditation, it is a matter of months or even years of working to improve your eyesight, not just a few weeks with the charts.

Once you are properly prepared through exercise, meditation, and a clear purpose, you will be ready to start observing human energy fields. What are the optimal conditions for seeing the aura? Some people claim that you can see the aura best in a dark room. The only thing you will see better under such conditions is the physical aura because that becomes translucent. But darkness absorbs the photons given off in the energy field, and therefore, the colors are really most visible against a white background. In the Philippines, there are several psychic surgeons who diagnose by observing the aura and who wrap their patients up in white sheets before they begin treatment. They do this because the aura becomes visible when reflected against the white sheet. Of course, it becomes confusing if the subject is standing directly in front of the light, as in front of a window, because then you do not know whether the light you see is shining from behind or whether it is part of the person's energy field.

In most cases, when people begin to see the energy fields around humans, they see the physical aura first because it is the densest. Generally, the next step is to start seeing rays because rays are most intense. Then they start seeing the subtler auric fields. It makes sense that the brighter colors would be seen first, with the subtler colors falling away into nothingness. When people say, "You've got a yellow aura," what they might actually be seeing is the ray. In such cases, they see it around the head and shoulders but never below.

When people come to the point where they can actually see auras well and are ready to begin interpreting them, I like to caution them about a few things, some of which I have said repeatedly in this book. First, we must realize that we are always looking through our own auras, and we must know our auras well in order to be able to distinguish them from what we see in the energy fields of others. Second, it is a good idea to inform the other person that we are not observing the aura as it occurs objectively, in its full and true nature, but that what we are observing of that person's aura depends on our own state of consciousness at that moment. Third, we should never tell people they have lived their lives wrong because they have not used the properties of the energy we have observed. We can only tell them what that energy is, mentioning the pros and cons and the areas where they may be vulnerable. Your disciplined practice may have improved your eyesight so that you are able to observe the ray and the aura, but that definitely does not put you in a position to tell anyone else what to do or not to do.

# 5 : The Naturopathic System of Energy Regulation

## Motion, the Law of Life

The basic law of life is motion, the rhythmic, cyclic pulsation of radiant energy. Not only is radiant energy found in the universe at large, but it is characteristic of all living things and of each of us individually. This is not a vague, invisible force out there in the cosmos; it is very real and tangible, for it exists in our bodies, in our clothing, and in the food we eat.

Science is now discovering that matter itself is made up of this energy, that beyond the molecule, beyond the atom, beyond the proton, the neutron, and the electron, there are components that can no longer be characterized as matter but can be considered either waves or particles, depending on the conditions under which they are observed. So from the viewpoint of quantum theory, all matter can be seen as a constant dance of energy; every particle of which we are composed is made up of these packets of radiant energy in constant motion.

Energy exists in four radical states: light, heat, moisture, and crystallization. We do not have to delve very far into esoteric writings to realize that these radical states of energy correspond to the four elements of the ancients: air, fire, water, and earth. Each of these states exhibits a different mode of energy flow, ranging from swift to slow, from free to bound; but all of them are nevertheless characterized by energy in constant motion. Even the densest matter, such as metal or stone, is in constant energetic motion.

Because the human body participates in this universal movement of energy, the four radical energy states must also be in evidence in the body. Indeed, the human body is designed for the transformation of energy, from its pure form as light, to its more solid, imprisoned form as fire, and then, through electrochemical transformations, into the increasingly dense forms of liquids and solids. And through a reversal of this process, through catabolism and elimination, solids are once again transformed into liquids, fire (heat), and light (as we have seen in Chapter 1).

## Health as Energy Flow

In order for energy to be transformed from one state to another, it must be in a constant flow through the body. We saw in Chapter 1 that the chakras, or energy centers, are the dynamos that provide the impetus for this flow. When a chakra's function is impeded or stagnated, this condition will be reflected in a decrease or distortion of its radiant output in the aura.

Any density in our makeup will hamper the flow of energy among our molecules. One way of looking at illness is to characterize it as stagnant energy, energy that is not being heightened and transformed.

We might compare our energy flow to the motion of a pendulum. At each end of the pendulum's swing, it has accumulated the kinetic power it needs to move back in the opposite direction. What happens when we hold onto energy? Let us say that one pole of the pendulum's swing is labeled "positive" and the other "negative." If we swing to the positive side and hold onto it, we are acting like goody-goodies who refuse to look at the negative because we think anything negative is bad. If we hold onto the positive side, we can never swing to the negative, and the energy of the pendulum becomes stagnant. There are other people who hang onto the negative, and the same thing happens; the pendulum never reaches the positive anymore, so there is an erratic rhythm. In your body, that means there is stagnation somewhere of the energies within you. In a healthy, active rhythm, the positive and negative are in a perfectly balanced state, which biologists call *homeostasis*. Ideally, we can go beyond the state of homeostasis; we do not really need to watch if things are positive or negative, whether our condition is hyper or hypo. When people are in such a rhythm, there is no positive and negative anymore, just a perpetual, mobile rhythm. Thus, the ideal is to achieve a perpetual motion so that you do not need to think about positive and negative any longer. As long as we still have to bring the positive together with the negative, we are actually trying to create a current. Once the current has been achieved, if you just let it go from then on and keep operating in that balanced state, you do not need to think in terms of positive and negative.

A healthy body is one whose elements are in balance. We have said that radiant energy is the basic building block of our bodies, as it is of the universe. This radiant energy, which pervades all matter, tends of itself to preserve its environment in balance and harmony through the principle of resonance (which we shall discuss in the next section). It is characteristic of this energy that it is progressive and evolutionary, pulsating from one state to the next. Sickness occurs when we inhibit this pulse, restrain our energy uncreatively, and resist the transitions through the natural stages of our lives. It is not always obvious what these natural stages are, but we can begin to attain a proper perspective when we realize that we cannot be alive and grow unless we can also die. Fear plays a large part in illness—fear of dying, of leaving behind one stage and entering the next. This fear restricts our flow of energy and stalls our growth. Our bodies are going through continuous changes every fraction of a second all during our lifetimes; these changes involve transformations, and this process of transformation, which is life, is also a process of dying.

An important aspect of balanced living, then, is balanced dying. As we take time out to eat and rest, we also need to take time out to die, to encourage the progressive transition of our selves through the stages of life. This time out for dying is how I think of meditation. That is the reason why the present volume, on health, follows the volume on meditation *(Voluntary Controls)*; meditation is the basic initiator of all action. Every emotional and mental action/thought immediately flows into physiological action. Thus, it is inevitable that heightened self-awareness will influence the body and will effect important changes on the physical level. It is only after we understand how these subtler influences can help us to maintain our health that we can truly understand the role of material aids in the process of preparing the body to heal itself.

## Assimilation Through Resonance

One way of looking at the mind-body spectrum is to say that energy is expressed in two formats: as pure energy, or spirit, and as matter. Pure energy is concerned with the causal side of our nature, and matter is spirit's material form of expression. These two states of energy are very closely related, which helps to explain how some few individuals have been able to sustain their bodies on very rarefied nourishment, on energy in its nearly pure state. If, through discipline and concentration, we were to allow our minds to operate fully in our bodies, we would so raise our transformational intensities that we could be nourished by more and more subtle forms of energy, leaving behind food as we know it altogether.

In dense, earthly forms, magnetism is a force whereby opposites attract; that is, positive attracts negative. But in the more rarefied realm of pure spirit, or mind, like attracts like. If we keep the body as radiant as possible, our higher consciousness will attract energy at that same high level, and so we will avoid diseases. On this high level of energy, which I call the *paramagnetic,* if we radiate out with a certain frequency of energy and with a certain amplitude, this will produce resonance with similar energies in the environment.

Resonance is reverberation. If I strike a G note on a violin and there is a piano three rooms away, that G note will travel through the air and set up a resonant vibration in the G string of the piano, which will then reverberate (inaudibly) back to the violin. The same thing is true of electromagnetic vibrations, which also have the capacity to resonate. Remember that all the particles you have in your body are also contained in the environment. Every particle has the capacity to produce an energetic outflow. (It is this electromagnetic outflow that is now being measured by sensitive devices such as the SQUID, described in Chapter 1.) Through this radiation coming from our bodies, then, we attract those particles that are equal in the frequency and amplitude of their vibration.

Most diseases can be characterized along a spectrum of sympathy and empathy. Sympathetic-type people live on an emotional level; they resonate only with dense and low pulsations, attracting energy that stagnates in their gut, thus causing disease. Empathy transforms this absorbed energy into a finer form, into light; and as it raises the amplitude of the energy, it will radiate out and be emitted, rather than stagnating.

For example, arthritis is a form of sympathetic illness. Arthritis in the body is usually matched by rigid thinking in the mind, and the latter is often the cause of the former. To cure arthritis requires that the body and the mind both become more flexible. Gold injections can sometimes increase physical flexibility, but such treatment should be accompanied by mental relaxation as well.

Obesity is also due to sympathy. Overweight people are sponges for everyone else's problems, for their random stagnant energy. Once absorbed, this dull energy settles in obese persons and does not move out again. Correspondingly, thoughts and feelings that do not get expressed and used will alter the body's chemistry, become dense, and turn into fat. Sympathy means "similar feeling," but empathy means "energy in motion with feeling." One secret of health is to raise gut feelings from the solar plexus level into the heart, where they can be transformed and expressed, radiated outward.

It is interesting that people who are thinkers and worriers, who are very sensitive to their environments, who attract all the sympathetic feelings and energies out of their environment quite often attract all kinds of particles to their bodies that become toxic to them. For example, we might look at numerous cases of skin conditions such as eczema, which dermatologists quite often have a very difficult time treating. They give the patients all kinds of tests and cannot find the cause of the skin condition; they may finally throw up their hands and say the skin problem is "psychosomatic."

I once treated a nine-year-old girl who would have an absolutely clear complexion when she went to school in the morning. She would be in class a half hour, and if somebody in the class had a headache or a sore toe or a sore throat, within that half an hour's time, the girl would have it, too. The way she then tried to get rid of it was by creating a poisonous substance in her body, which would cause her whole body to break out suddenly in eczema. She had to be taught to have her energy flowing before she went to school so that she would have a good electrical field around her and would not pick up any of the lower things in her environment.

These lower energies and toxic substances are all around us, but the only way we can be attracted to them is if we become electromagnetically sympathetic to them, if we let our energy go down. Doctors of course refer to this condition as having a "low resistance level"; they should also call it a *low consciousness level* because consciousness means energy. When you expand your consciousness, you are expanding your energy. If you have a low resistance because you have a low consciousness, your immunity factor goes downhill. (Note that the immunity mechanism is centered in the thymus gland, which is the gland associated with the heart chakra, the seat of consciousness.) This is why you have to find excitement and joy in all the things you do.

You can create this excitement within you. It is very valuable to realize that you can even use anger to create this excitement if you do not allow the anger to clot up in your solar plexus, where it will start to backfire on you. When you get angry, express the emotion in a creative act, not by boxing your children on the ears. You can clean out your closet or your desk, shine your shoes or brush your clothes, dig in your garden. You may be muttering about that so-and-so the whole time, but if you use that anger, the energy will then be beneficial for you. It is not wasted, and it does not affect you in the solar plexus area; rather, it creates an energy field around you. This is a very important lesson for our modern world, in which we are subjected to so many sources of frustration and anger. Some yogis use this tool when they go out into the desert and have nothing to get angry about anymore but need extra energy for their meditation. They may see a fly or some other insect buzzing around them, and they appear to get terribly mad, yelling, "What is this insect doing in my environment? I'm going to catch it!" Through all their excitement, they suddenly feel charged up by the power, and they go into meditation with new energy.

Society has taught us that we must control our anger. But we have never understood the meaning of control; we always think of control as suppression or repression, rather than as letting the energy flow. Power, which is another word for control, is a very valuable thing; but we use it wrongly, if not to repress ourselves, then to repress the rest of the world with it. So, if you have anger, do not repress it, but bring it out in a powerful action. That does not mean you have to knock somebody over. There are plenty of things that need to be done that you can do with the energy from your anger.

What I am saying is that the energy we radiate is crucial in determining what we attract to ourselves. This principle of resonance underlies the approach I take to healing and nutrition. Every particle of matter vibrates at a certain rate peculiar to itself. Through the process of assimilation, the body attracts to itself the elements it needs to grow and survive.

The world around us contains all the nutrients we require for a healthy and balanced life. Quite often, we do not choose what is suitable for our growth and balanced maintenance; but even if we were to eat the right foods, we might still remain unhealthy because of poor assimilation. Chemical, nutritional, or vitamin deficiencies—whatever you might call such causes of ill health—cannot be overcome merely by filling the organism with all of its missing elements and nutrients. If the organism is not capable of absorbing these aids, it cannot regain balanced functioning, which is health.

The body ingests nourishment in a heavy form because the body is heavy. A more subtle body assimilates finer energy. But the body has the potential and the task of transforming the energy it ingests into more subtle energy. We are not bound to the heaviness of our organisms, for we have the capacity to transform the energy within ourselves into finer and finer levels. We assimilate our nourishment from meat and spinach and eggs because we already share an affinity for the energy in these substances. When they are assimilated into our organism, these substances assume a finer form and are put to more subtle uses. Assimilation is just another word for resonance; the body assimilates more effectively as it resonates in rhythm with the more subtle energetic pulses of the universe. This is our natural birthright, and so we are responsible if we abuse this right and cut ourselves off from the finer nourishment, or energy, surrounding us.

The proper approach to nutrition starts when we analyze our deficiencies and then prepare the body to satisfy its needs naturally from the world around it. The atmosphere and a reasonable diet are enough to provide all our needs if the body is working at peak efficiency. You should not need to take vitamin or mineral supplements all your life; once an imbalance is identified, the body can be prepared to assimilate its needs and then given these needs in the form of a dietary supplement. Thereafter, the body can recover its own balance and maintain itself in health with no further external assistance.

Let us now see how the body maintains this balance and how we prepare ourselves organically for autonomous health.

## Ions and Electromagnetic Energy Regulation

We have already said that through electrochemical reactions within the body, there is a continuous transformation from chemistry into energy and from energy back into chemistry. How does this energy become available to the body, and how does it undergo such transmutations? The exchange of energy in our bodies takes place through the exchange of *ions*, which are simply components of molecules, either atoms or groups of atoms, that have lost or taken on electrons and hence have an electric charge.

The molecules of which our bodies are composed are actually built up and broken down through the exchange of ions. The affinities that unite these two spheres of life, the ionic and the molecular, are really only extensions of that invisible activity that pervades the universe, the electromagnetic forces radiating in all directions.

Our bodies are composed for the most part of water. The processes of this mass of water, which flows through our body, are of the utmost importance because the body fluids act as a catalyst, carrying and adjusting all external influences and nutrition throughout every part of the body. Furthermore, the paramagnetic quality of our body fluids (like attracting like) depends on a constant process of the creation and combination of ions in this fluid, on the ionic balance between positive and negative.

To make changes in the body, then, means to change the electromagnetic state of the body's fluid. Electricity is the particular characteristic of the energy force we are dealing with, and magnetism is the direction given to that force. Disease, old age, and other alterations in the body's energy patterns are ultimately traceable to imbalances and declines in the electrical potency of the body plasma, its intermolecular fluid.

In its function as a catalyst, it is important that our body fluid conduct electrochemical energy in just the right way. If our water were just a conductor pure and simple, that would mean that any electrical energy contained in it would be dissipated, distributed out. A good conductor, without insulation, cannot retain any energy in it, and the energy in such a fluid would simply disappear over a period of time. Our body fluid must be electrochemically balanced so that it can conduct energy without losing it; it should be dielectric water. Distilled water is perfectly neutral in this sense, which means that it can latch onto all chemicals and nutrients and charges and retain them.

In this connection, we might look at the current popularity of water beds. People get very excited about sleeping on water beds, but they often complain that they are terribly tired. They do not realize that they have opened all the gates of their energies because the water in the water bed is tap water, which is so chemically unbalanced that it is conductive, meaning that all the energies go through it and dissipate. All the psychic energy, all the thought patterns, all the electrical messages—everything moves through the water and is lost. This may affect your mental state; you may have terrible subconscious dreams on a water bed because there is no insulation, and you start to let your own energy leak out.

This condition is what I call a *bleeding aura.* It can also result from a lack of the proper electrochemical insulation in the body's fluids, and it is elements such as calcium that provide this insulation in our bodies. So if you want to sleep on a water bed, that's fine, as long as you go to the extra trouble and expense of filling it with distilled water. Then it is not conductive anymore; it is dielectric. Then your energies will not be dissipated during the night.

## Elements and Cell Salts

The basic chemical elements are those substances we need to subsist in good health. In the normal gross fashion in which our bodies function, we derive nourishment from energy in molecular form, or food. Yet, what the body is really doing to obtain nourishment is to assimilate the basic ionic vibrations of the particular elements that it needs and that exist in various foods. My program of health and nutrition is therefore concerned with bringing the body into a state in which it is able to assimilate, break down, and extract the nutrition it requires.

Let me provide an example of assimilation. If my body needs the element silicon, I eat a cucumber, which contains silicon. But how does the cucumber's silicon get assimilated by my body's fluid substance, which is where the silicon will be most effective? Absorption is not certain enough, for absorption refers only to the molecular process; and now that we know we must focus on the ionic level, we want to encourage another process, which is resonance. Like attracts like in ionic electromagnetism, so attraction and assimilation are accomplished when the ionic resonance of silicon is matched by the resonance of the body fluid. But the body fluid will only radiate with the pulse of silicon when the fluid already contains enough of the element silicon to make it so resonate. That is, if the body fluid is to extract the silicon contained in the cucumber, there have to be silicon ions already in the body fluid. So, if there is a serious silicon deficiency in the body, eating cucumbers will not solve it because the body cannot properly assimilate its silicon.

The cell salts, of which there are twelve, are a special class of homeopathically prepared chemical compounds, each consisting of an electropositive and an electronegative component, or ion, that have been subjected to a special process of dilution to make these elements more readily available to the body. This employment of elements in combination (such as sodium with phosphorus) is designed to anticipate the body's mode of extracting what it requires of sodium or of phosphorus. In the case of these two elements, for example, the phosphorus is in the form of phosphate. In isolation, as pure elements, the sodium and the phosphorus may be difficult to assimilate; but in order to be combined into a salt, they must already be in ionic form, and thus they help each other to be assimilated.

If the body requires an energy supplement, it will not do any good to stuff the organism with only a positively charged ion. The body, as a bipolar electrical energy field, requires both poles to be activated. So, an energy supplement should contain both a positively charged element, such as iron, and an equal amount of a negatively charged element, such as phosphorus. These nutrients can be put into the organism in the form in which they have been assimilated by other living things, in plants and animal tissues rich in iron and phosphorus, or in a diluted form, in a cell salt.

The *cell salts* are so named because they represent levels of dilution approaching the concentration of these substances in the cells themselves. When I say the cell salts are diluted, I do not necessarily mean they are watered down; on the contrary, a high energy is obtained through dilution. In the preparation of cell salts, the dilution process consists of repeated trituration, which is the painstaking grinding of the chemical compound, or salt, in a mortar and pestle together with a substance that is electrochemically neutral and that is capable of taking the impression of the electrically charged ions of the salt, insulating it, and holding it. Lactose, or milk sugar, is such a substance; it will retain the electrical potential of the cell salt until it is released by being put into a fluid. This is the reason for never taking cell salts diluted in water or even in the hand; as soon as they come into contact with moisture, they lose their charge, or potency, before they have a chance to enter the body.

The process of trituration is a process of serial dilution of the salt with lactose, in the ratio of 1 part of the salt to 9 parts of lactose, or a 1:10 dilution. After the original 1:10 dilution has been meticulously prepared by long grinding together of the substances, 1 part of this mixture is triturated with another 9 parts of lactose to produce a 1:100 dilution. The process is repeated until the desired dilution, or potency, is obtained. Common potencies for cell salts are $3x$, which means 1 part in $10^3$, or 1:1,000; $6x$, or $10^6$, which is equal to 1:1,000,000; and $12x$, or $10^{12}$, which is the same as a 1:1,000,000,000,000 dilution. This does not mean that the less diluted form, or lower potency, is necessarily stronger. Less diluted also means denser, and the denser the material, the longer it takes to be assimilated; whereas the more diluted form is more quickly assimilated and thus stirs up the system more. Thus, the $3x$ strength, a relatively low potency or low dilution, is suitable for slow building up, as with magnesium phosphate, when a higher potency (or higher dilution) might be too much of a shock to the system; whereas $6x$ is appropriate for instances in which prompter action is necessary.

Whereas the cell salts assist the anabolic, or building-up, processes in the body, the elements control the catabolic, or breaking-down, processes. Together, these processes constitute metabolism. So, metabolism is really an expression of the dual acts of conservation and distribution of vital energy throughout the body, which are the work of the cell salts (conservation) and the elements (distribution).

The many minerals and trace elements are the specific forms in which the four basic elements of the ancients (earth, water, fire, and air) are found on our planet. Despite their sometimes dense appearance, the elements all function within living organisms to encourage the movement, or distribution, of energy. Trace elements are so called because only the merest traces of these substances are found throughout the body and especially in the glands associated with the seven chakras. The minerals, in contrast, are found in relatively large quantities; some of them are among the basic building blocks of the body. However, whether the minerals and trace elements exist in large or infinitesimal quantities in the body, they all appear to be vital to the maintenance of the healthy, balanced functioning of the organism.

Although our bodies contain aspects of all the organic life forms on our planet, they are also unable to exist without inorganic foundations, the elements. All organic processes are bound up with the inorganic activities in the cell, which holds in balance the relationship between the salts and the elements.

The cell salts represent the usual structures that condense, insulate, and transmit the ionized potency of the basic elements from their raw state, through the body's digestive process, and finally into the body fluid. The cell salts thus aid in the distribution of the elements throughout the body.

Cell salts are compounds, and like all chemical compounds, they represent imprisoned potential energy awaiting release. The purpose of cell salts is to produce stability by integrating and utilizing the energies of the elements, through centripetal, or inward-drawing, forces.

In contrast, the elements are the centrifugal, or outward-moving, forces that distribute radiant energy throughout the body in waves and whorls, horizontal and vertical waves; these create vortices, the radiant patterns that, as we have seen, are the characteristic feature of the aura.

The ions of dissolved salts regulate metabolism, and in this way, the salts balance the centrifugal radiance of the elements. This balance is very tenuous; the slightest imbalance in the fluid chemistry will have wide repercussions in the entire organism. The minerals and trace elements must be in proper balance in our bodies if they are to fulfill their role of distributing energy. If they are out of balance, they are not able to trigger the energy and keep it flowing. For example, if a person has a potassium deficiency, there is automatically also excessive sodium content in the body. Such an imbalance is like a short circuit in our energy pattern; that is why we need to adjust such imbalances by the use of cell salts.

Table 3 lists some of the important elements and minerals. In their free states, each of these elements has a certain set of qualities and is associated with a certain wavelength. This is the basis for what I call the *selective affinities* (to which I refer in Chapter 6). When these elements are combined with each other to form a salt, the resulting compound has new characteristics that may differ from the original elements. Table 3 describes the elements in their free states, along with what makes each of them important for the body. The description of a cell salt in Table 4 may be quite different from those of the two elements of which it is formed.

## Instructions for Taking Cell Salts

The purpose of maintaining the proper cell salt balance in the body is to attract and extract the mineral elements we need from our regular diet. Under ordinary circumstances, the cell salts themselves should also be readily extracted from our diet. But to counteract specific deficiencies, it is appropriate to stimulate the process of assimilation by taking the extracted cell salts in tablet form.

Because cell salts are among the least potentially detrimental dietary supplements you can take, it is safe to experiment on yourself with them. After analyzing your needs and possible deficiencies by studying Table 4 and also perhaps following the suggestions for your tarot card (see Chapter 6), you may select one or more cell salts to try. A normal dosage would be sixteen tablets per day, either four tablets four times during the day or eight tablets twice a day, in the morning and in the evening.

Because these cell salts have an electrical potential, it is very important to take them dry with a spoon and never to touch them with your hands. The moisture on your skin is ionized and would neutralize the potency of the tablets; that is, your own body moisture would literally de-charge the cell salts. You can also just pour the indicated number of tablets into the bottle cap and then directly into your mouth. As I noted earlier, never take the tablets with water; just let them dissolve under your tongue. Keep the bottle tightly closed and away from moisture, heat, light, and other medicinal substances.

If you begin taking a specific cell salt for a specific ailment, do so for a few months, and then stop. The body should have been able in that time to make up its deficiency, and you should see some improvement in your body's ability to assimilate its requirements, as evidenced by a lessening of your deficiency symptoms. Thereafter, you may take Bio-plasma, which is a balanced maintenance combination of cell salts. If you see no improvement in your condition after taking the cell salt, you will need to analyze your eating habits and your way of living more carefully to ascertain what may be preventing the cell salt treatment from taking effect.

**TABLE 3: SOME IMPORTANT MINERALS AND TRACE ELEMENTS**

| Element | Electric Charge | Description and Function | Organs Requiring | Dietary Sources |
|---|---|---|---|---|
| Calcium | electropositive (alkali forming) | A metallic substance found in alkaline earth, such as lime and chalk; a base for plaster of paris. Calcium solidifies and crystallizes and therefore acts as an integrator, a building block. For the nervous system, it acts as an insulator. Its utility is not limited to bones. Calcification in the body can be broken up with calcium in ionic form, which will spread the calcium to other parts of the body, thereby breaking up calcium crystallization (see *silicon*). | adrenal cortex, muscles, nails, ovaries, prostate, skeleton, skin, teeth, thymus | almonds, Brazil nuts, citrus peel, filbert nuts, green vegetables, leaves of herbs and plants, milk, seaweed, sesame seeds, sunflower seeds |
| Chlorine | electronegative (acid forming) | A greenish yellow gas, two and a half times heavier than air, and very soluble in water, so it is fast-acting in solution; poisonous in gas form. Essential for the formation of hydrochloric acid, releasing oxygen in the process. Hydrochloric acid is needed for digestion and for the brain. | hair, intestines, liver, muscles, pancreas, skin, spleen, teeth, thyroid | avocado, celery, coconut, dates, kale, kelp, lettuce, tomato, turnip |
| Copper | electropositive (alkali forming) | A reddish brown, malleable, and ductile metal that is an excellent conductor of electricity and heat. Essential for utilization of iron in the diet. Highly concentrated in pineal gland. However, too much copper can make you sluggish. | blood, brain, liver, pancreas | apricots, beans (especially pinto beans), nuts, whole grains |

| | | | |
|---|---|---|---|
| Fluorine | A yellowish green gas, corrosive, poisonous; the most highly reactive element known. Attacks and destroys organic substances. An excess can cause spinal and bone diseases. | electronegative (acid forming) | adrenal cortex, brain, eyes, ovaries, prostate, teeth, thymus | almonds, beet greens, carrots, dandelion greens, spinach, turnip greens |
| Iodine | A nonmetallic element in the same family as chlorine and fluorine, consisting of grayish black, volatile crystals that form a violet-colored vapor. Essential to the synthesis of thyroid hormones. Deficiency can lead to goiter. | electronegative (acid forming) | adrenal medulla, hair, pineal, pituitary, thyroid | asparagus, blueberries, dulse, Irish moss, kale, kelp, all seafood (especially shellfish), spinach, Swiss chard, turnip greens, watermelon |
| Iron | Occurs in nature as a metallic ore, that is, a mineral mixed with a metal, from which the metal is extracted. It is essential for the formation of hemoglobin, and in combination with potassium, it is a carrier of oxygen. An excellent healing agent. As iron phosphate (FERRUM-PHOS), it can raise blood pressure, so must be used with caution. | neutral (catalyst) | adrenal cortex, blood, brain, heart, kidneys, muscles, ovaries, prostate, skin, thymus | cayenne pepper, dulse, green vegetable leaves, kelp, squash, wines (port and sherry; wines are a suitable way for older persons to acquire easily assimilated iron) |
| Magnesium | A silver white metal, hard and light. It burns very brightly. General distributor of other elements in the organism. Restores the current of energy in blood and nerves. Deficiency may cause weakness, depression, disturbances in muscle contraction. | electropositive (alkali forming) | adrenals, brain, intestines, kidneys, liver, pancreas, spleen, thyroid | almonds, bananas, beans, dates, dried fruit (nonsulfurized only) all greens, kelp, potatoes |
| Manganese | A grayish white metal, usually hard and brittle. Rusts like iron but is not magnetic. | neutral (catalyst) | adrenal medulla, brain, eyes, pineal, pituitary | beets, carrots, celery, chives, cucumbers, parsley |

TABLE 3: SOME IMPORTANT MINERALS AND TRACE ELEMENTS (Continued)

| Element | Electric Charge | Description and Function | Organs Requiring | Dietary Sources |
|---|---|---|---|---|
| Phosphorus | electronegative (acid forming) | A white and waxy solid, becoming yellow when exposed to light. When exposed to air, it gives off white fumes and an odor of garlic. It can be very poisonous, but as an ingredient of myelin, it acts as a protective agent for muscular tissue and for nerves. Aids in the proper assimilation of calcium and magnesium. | adrenal medulla, brain, hair, heart, pineal, pituitary | beans (legumes), dried fruit (nonsulfurized only), all grains, green vegetable leaves, nuts, seaweed, all seeds |
| Potassium | electropositive (alkali forming) | A silver white substance that easily unites with oxygen; it decomposes in water, producing a slight explosion and flame. Crucial in maintaining balance in the nervous system. In each nerve cell, the center should be filled with potassium ions, the membrane with sodium ions, and the structure solidified with calcium and silicon. Also produces and regulates body heat. | heart, liver, muscles, pancreas, spleen, stomach and digestive tract, thyroid | avocado, bananas, beans (legumes), beets, carrots, dried fruit (nonsulfurized), green vegetable leaves, nuts, radishes, seaweed |
| Silicon | electronegative (acid forming) | Found in rock crystals, such as quartz and flint; a very hard substance; found in mineral springs. It not only promotes firmness and strength in the organism but also radiates energy. It can form itself into a wide variety of crystal forms. Citrus acid eats away the calcium covering the bones; liver oils will relubricate dried bones; and silicon (as an elasticizer) with calcium will restore bones. Healing properties; integrates and stabilizes; cuts away putrid matter. | adrenal cortex, brain, eyes, hair, heart, ovaries, prostate, skin, teeth, thymus | avocado, cucumbers, dandelions, lettuce, shave grass, strawberries, sunflower seeds |

| | | | | |
|---|---|---|---|---|
| Sodium | electropositive (alkali forming) | A soft, silver white, waxy, metallic substance. It has a great affinity for water; it floats on the surface and gradually disappears with a hissing noise, indicating that hydrogen is being given off, forming caustic soda. All sodium should be kept well sealed to prevent access to air. Predominant in the intracellular fluid. In excess, can cause edema. | gallbladder, intestines, liver, nails, pancreas, skeleton, skin, spleen, stomach and digestive tract, teeth, thyroid | beets (roots and greens), carrots, celery, dried fruit (nonsulfurized), kale, kelp, radishes, raisins |
| Sulfur | electronegative (acid forming) | A solid crystal, greenish gray, with a faint odor and taste. Although it fuses and boils, it is insoluble in water. It burns with a blue flame when united with oxygen. | adrenal medulla eyes, hair, nails, pituitary, skeleton, skin, stomach and digestive tract, teeth | kale, kelp, lettuce, raspberries, turnips |
| Zinc | electropositive (alkali forming) | A bluish white metal. Highly concentrated in the pineal gland. | hair | celery, lettuce, sunflower seeds, wheat germ |

## A Survey of the Cell Salts

The three principal electropositive elements that are attracted to the body and from which the cell salts are formed are sodium, potassium, and calcium.

Sodium, or natrium (Na), has a strong affinity·for water, and so it is a potent distributor of fluids throughout the body.

Potassium, or kalium (K), has a tendency to unite with oxygen to produce heat and fire, and so it is an important element in producing and regulating body temperature.

Calcium, or calcarea (Ca), has the chief properties of integration, solidification, and crystallization; it is therefore an important building block of body tissues.

The cell salts may be organized into four *biotonic classes,* based on their function within the body, as follows:

*Shifting, or sulfur, group.* This group stirs up and shifts waste matter, aiding detoxification; it includes sodium sulfate, potassium sulfate, and calcium sulfate.

*Eliminating, or chlorine, group.* This group encourages efficient elimination of putrid matter. This recuperative function suitably follows the cleansing function of the first group. This group includes sodium chloride, potassium chloride, and sodium phosphate.

*Binding, or calcium, group.* This group promotes the integration of matter and the building up of new matter. It includes calcium sulfate, calcium fluoride, and iron phosphate.

*Distributing, or phosphorus, group.* This group, which controls molecular balance and the rhythms of the healthy organism, includes potassium phosphate, magnesium phosphate, and silicea.

Table 4 indicates the principal functions of each of the cell salts, as well as the conditions that may indicate a deficiency or imbalance of that cell salt in the body. On the basis of these descriptions, you may be able to ascertain which of the cell salts you may need to restore a healthy balance in the functioning of your body.

## An Introduction to the Use of Herbs

Herbs are. once again becoming an increasingly popular means of treating illness. These medicinal plants not only act in a remedial manner but also help to keep the energy flowing.

Appendix A lists many common medicinal herbs and their therapeutic applications. Medicinal herbs should not be taken on a daily-mainte-

## TABLE 4: THE CELL SALTS

---

**SULFUR, OR SHIFTING, GROUP**

*Calcium phosphate (calcarea phosphorica, calc-phos, $Ca_3(PO_4)_2$)* *

This cell salt acts like mortar in the body, integrating all the body's tissues. It is found in all the tissues of the body, is essential to the sound formation of bone and proper growth, and is a vital element in all the functions of nutrition and assimilation. Checks dehydration and violent elimination processes; controls solidifying activities, and prevents them from becoming extreme. Deficiency conditions include bone diseases, defective nutrition, poor teeth, weakness, emaciation, digestive disturbances, slow growth in children, delayed teething. A general nutrient for simple anemia, debility, and impaired digestion. Especially valuable in old people for its restorative powers after acute illness.

*Potassium sulfate (kalium sulphuricum, kali-sulph, $K_2SO_4$)*

Promotes the formation of oils in the body; softens and lubricates tissues, breaks up solid deposits, keeps the pores open, ejects oil, and encourages perspiration. This salt has a great affinity for the skin and mucous membranes, acting both as a lubricant and as a healer through its promotion of oil secretions. Good for minor skin eruptions, bronchial catarrh. Disturbances of the balance of this cell salt are characterized by yellowish, slimy secretions, yellow-coated tongue; indigestion; secretions from eyes, ears, and nose with characteristic yellowish color. Also excellent for calcium deposits (in combination with silicea).

*Sodium sulfate (natrum sulphuricum, natrum-sulph, $Na_2SO_4$)*

This salt is not a constituent of cells; it is found only in the intercellular fluid. It influences the excretion of superfluous water by attracting and extracting fluid from the organism; it stirs up and shifts body fluids during the process of digestion, elimination, and respiration. For this reason, NATRUM-SULPH is added to some diuretics. This salt is especially attracted to the intestinal and abdominal regions. It is excellent for bilious conditions with such symptoms as greenish brown coated root of tongue, bitter taste, colic, and so on, for liver problems, and to counter influenza.

**CHLORINE, OR ELIMINATING, GROUP**

*Potassium chloride (kalium muriaticum, kali-mur, KCl)*

Distributes oxygen throughout the body, promoting oxygenation of the organism and thus assisting in the elimination of waste matter. Stirs up organic energy, and awakens dormant life forces; acts as an antidepressant as it creates and moves energy; can create real explosions of energy. The metabolic function of KALI-MUR is to unite with albumin to form fibrin. When this cell salt is not in proper balance, albumin is released in the form of thick, white, sticky discharges from the skin or mucous membranes, white or gray-coated tongue. A good blood conditioner, for use against cough, colds, respiratory ailments; follows FERRUM-PHOS when excretions set in from the affected parts.

## TABLE 4: THE CELL SALTS

---

### CHLORINE, OR ELIMINATING, GROUP

#### Sodium chloride (natrum muriaticum, nat-mur, NaCl)

This salt is a constituent of every liquid and hence of every solid in the body. The body is about 70 percent water, and Natrum Mur regulates the proper utilization of water and the degree of moisture in the cells. It attracts water from without, taking up moisture from the atmosphere and thereby helping the body to adapt to atmospheric changes. It also helps to extract and stabilize fluids from foods. A deficiency of this salt may cause the water to remain in the intercellular fluids, leading to bloating and profuse watery secretions. Deficiency may also cause dryness and loss of smell and taste.

#### Sodium phosphate (natrum phosphoricum, nat-phos, $Na_3PO_4$)

Regulates the alkaline-acid balance of the body. As an alkalizer, it decomposes and emulsifies fatty tissue. Useful in diets to prevent fat from settling in one place. Also used as an acid neutralizer for conditions of excess acidity, digestive upsets, heartburn, yellowish itching secretions from skin or membranes, tongue with creamy yellow coating, stomach and intestinal disturbances.

### CALCIUM, OR BINDING, GROUP

#### Calcium fluoride (calcarea fluorata, calc-fluor, $CaF_2$)

This cell salt is a constituent of the elastic fibers of the skin, connective tissue, and blood vessels, as well as being found in the glands, bones, and tooth enamel. It solidifies and crystallizes fluids, binding colloidal substances. A nonconductor of nerve energy, it insulates the nerve cells and helps protect the organism from overstrain. Indicated in conditions of dilated, relaxed blood vessels or elastic tissues such as varicose veins, impaired circulation, hemorrhoids; muscular weakness; hard or swollen glands. Prevents nails and hair from becoming brittle.

#### Calcium sulfate (calcarea sulphurica, calc-sulph, $CaSO_4$)

This salt's function is to destroy worn-out red blood cells, thereby promoting their elimination from the body. It lines the blood vessels and is extremely absorbent; it absorbs diseased cells and bacteria, covers and protects all soft tissues from deterioration and injury. Impaired function of this cell salt will produce symptoms such as catarrh, skin disorders, ulceration, boils, respiratory ailments, unhealthy skin, slow-healing minor injuries, thick, yellowish, offensive secretions. It is a blood purifier that will help clear up minor skin irritations, acne, and pimples; assists slow-healing wounds.

#### Iron phosphate (ferrum phosphoricum, fer-phos, $FePO_4$)

A constituent of the hemoglobin in red blood cells, this cell salt controls the formation of hemoglobin and the distribution of oxygen through the blood to the body. This combination of iron with phosphorus can raise blood pressure, so it must be taken with caution. A deficiency can produce symptoms of anemia, leading to fever and inflammation. An especially good cell salt for children, especially for sniffles, colds, and anemia. Indicated in the early stages of most ailments characterized by fever, inflammation, heat, and pain, especially before secretions from the affected part set in.

**PHOSPHORUS, OR DISTRIBUTING, GROUP**

*Magnesium phosphate (magnesium phosphoricum, mag-phos, $Mg_3(PO_4)_2$)*

This cell salt is composed of two light-producing elements: magnesium, which is capable of spreading out in long, thin threads and which burns with a brilliant light, and phosphorus, which emits light spontaneously. MAG-PHOS is essential to the metabolic processes of the nerve and muscle fibers of the body. The light-producing powers of its component elements make it an excellent distributor of energy throughout the body. Its radiating qualities make it able to cut across fibers and disperse tangled knots of tension, as in the abdominal plexi or the hypogastric gland. An excellent distributor of vital energy throughout the organism; restores normal body rhythm. Deficiency of this salt is marked by muscular fiber contractions, painful spasms of the nerves and muscles. Characteristic symptoms of deficiency are sharp, darting spasmodic pains, neuralgic pains in any part of the body. In various nerve disorders, the use of MAG-PHOS in alternation with KALI-PHOS is usually very desirable.

*Potassium phosphate (kali phosphoricum, kali-phos, $K_3PO_4$)*

A constituent of the tissues of nerves, brain, and muscles, as well as of blood cells, this salt combines the elements of air and fire. It stimulates the nerve fibers and awakens the protoplasmic activity in the cells. This is the basic salt for brain tissues and nerve fluids. It unclogs the flow of energy, giving a lively, tingling feeling to the body. It is the most radioactive of all the cell salts, as well as having a tendency to unite with carbon. This cell salt, which is lacking in many individuals, is a stimulating salt, awakening the activity of the whole substantial self. Deficiency symptoms include mental weakness, depression, irritability, nervousness, sometimes general debility, neuralgic pains. This cell salt is often used to counter nervous indigestion and nervous headache.

*Silicea (silica, silicic oxide, $SiO_2$)*

This oxide of silicon is the only cell salt that is not a double salt, composed of two mineral elements. Silicea is an integral part of the structure of plants and to a lesser extent of animals and humans. It can assume a variety of crystalline formations and so imparts strength and integration to the body. It is a constituent of bones, joints, glands, skin, and mucous surfaces. Silicea functions as an electrical insulator and purifies the system by controlling the normal molecular flow, keeping the organism in rhythmic balance. It gives firmness and vibrancy to the nerves and tissues. It exerts a cleansing and healing action. Symptoms calling for silicea include catarrhal conditions of the respiratory organs with offensive, puslike discharges, offensive characteristic secretions, skin eruptions with offensive discharges, suppurative conditions that are slow to heal, small wounds that are slow to heal.

---

*The first listing for each entry is the English name; next, in parentheses, is the Latin version, followed by the abbreviation used by pharmacists.

nance basis; rather, they should be used as specific remedies when something goes wrong with your body. It is all right to drink herb teas as refreshing beverages, but in that case, avoid using the same herb all the time, or you will get a medicinal effect.

When I give herbs for medicinal purposes, I very rarely give single herbs; rather, I give them in combination. The most important herb in such a combination is the *curative,* which is the one that is selected for its medicinal effect on the specific condition being treated. This one curative may have such a strong action on the body that it is best to tone it down. That is why I give another herb, a *demulcent,* which softens the harshness of the curative. I also give an *aromatic,* which imparts fragrance and flavor to the herbal tea. Sometimes, I add a fourth herb, which serves as an activator or a tonic, to reinforce the curative. The type of activator I personally prefer to give would be a *laxative,* to make sure that we start removing some of the morbid matter through the intestinal tract.

If you refer to Appendix A, you will find that there are a number of herbs listed as demulcents, aromatics, and laxatives. After you have selected the curative for the specific therapeutic action you need, you can then choose the demulcent, aromatic, and laxative according to what you feel is suitable in each particular case.

In preparing an herbal tea, the curative should be twice the dosage of the other herbs. If we say that 1/2 teaspoon is equal to 1 part, then the curative would be 2 parts, or 1 teaspoon. For 1 quart of water, the component herbs should be in the following proportions:

| | | | |
|---|---|---|---|
| Curative | 2 parts | = | 1 teaspoon |
| Demulcent | 1 part | = | 1/2 teaspoon |
| Aromatic | 1 part | = | 1/2 teaspoon |
| Laxative (optional) | 1 part | = | 1/2 teaspoon |

Unless you are directed otherwise under the listing for a particular herb, never boil your herbs with the water. The few herbs that are boiled are the exception. Boil the water first, as for regular tea. Add the herbs in the indicated proportions, steep the mixture for ten to fifteen minutes, and serve the tea by the cup. You should not boil the herbs with the water because you may begin to extract chemicals in the boiling process that will act unpredictably on you or will interact with each other. If you simply add freshly boiled water to the herbs, the heat of the boiled water will be sufficient to draw out the medicinal ingredients. Ten to fifteen minutes is just the amount of time it takes to draw out the medicinal virtues of the herbs.

To illustrate the use of Appendix A and the formula for blended teas, let us say that you are suffering from nervousness and headache. As a curative, you will want an herb for your nerves, so you look under "Nervines." Valerian is a good choice as a nervine, so you can use 1 teaspoon of Valerian as a curative.

Now you must select a demulcent, an aromatic, and optionally, a laxative. There is no particular pattern to these supplementary herbs; for example, certain aromatics do not necessarily go with certain curatives. This is a matter of personal taste. But if you can find an aromatic or a demulcent that has the same application as the curative, as well as its supplementary function, then you would pick such an herb to help the curative's action. When you look under "Aromatics," for example, you will find chamomile; checking under "Chamomile" in Part 2 of Appendix A, you will find that chamomile is a nervine as well as an aromatic. It is logical, then, that you would prefer chamomile as an aromatic above one that has nothing to do with calming the nerves. But it is up to you to make the choice; it is not really that important.

You may find, then, that an herb fills a double function. If your purpose is to get rid of a headache and calm your nerves, you have a double effect from chamomile as an aromatic because it also reinforces the calmative action of the valerian. We need a demulcent, too. Licorice root is listed under "Demulcents" in Part I, but in Part II, you will find that it is also a laxative. It would make no sense, then, in this particular case to add a fourth herb. The licorice root can function both as a demulcent and as a laxative.

Our recipe for the herbal tea for nervousness and headache would then be:

> 1 quart water, boiled
> 1 teaspoon valerian root (curative)
> 1/2 teaspoon chamomile (aromatic)
> 1/2 teaspoon licorice root (demulcent and laxative)
>
> Add boiled water to the herbs, steep for 10 to 15 minutes, and drink one cup at a time.

People also use herbs as flavoring agents in cooking. There is no reason why you should not do this, of course, but be prepared for any medicinal effect such herbs may have. For example, you can make a nice licorice ice cream or licorice pudding, but if you put a lot of licorice root in your food, do not be surprised if you find yourself making a lot of trips to the bathroom; licorice can be a very strong laxative.

Some herbs you would never think of using in cooking because they have a bad taste. For example, you would never put valerian root in a salad because it has a nasty, bitter taste. This is the reason we use the aromatic in herbal teas: to take away the harshness of the flavor of the curative, to make it more palatable.

This brief introduction should enable you to make use of the information on herbs in Appendix A. One warning is in order: Note that some herbs are marked with an asterisk (*). As noted in the introduction to Appendix A, these herbs are toxic in one way or another and should be avoided if possible; in any case, they should only be used under the conditions described in the introduction to the appendix.

## Some Observations on Diet

The elements from the earth's crust are an excellent source of energy. Table 3 describes some dietary sources of important minerals and trace elements. Remember, however, that your body must be able to assimilate these elements from your food if your diet is to do you any good. Therefore, if you are eating the proper, balanced diet and still show deficiency symptoms, you might look into the use of cell salts to prepare your body to assimilate nutrients properly.

In general, root vegetables have a much higher mineral and trace element content than plants that grow above the soil. Red beets, for example, are a tremendous source of energy. Plants grown in volcanic soil and seaweeds, such as dulse and kelp, are also very rich sources of nutrients.

For those people who want to avoid eating meat, a vegetarian diet is perfectly capable of providing the body with its nutrients, but one must remember to diversify the vegetarian cuisine with plenty of non-green vegetables. Sometimes vegetarians look lethargic and mentally dull, which may be because they are taking in excessive quantities of green vegetables, which have a tendency to relax and dull the organism. Vital energy is much more concentrated in pigmented vegetables, such as red cabbage, beets, parsnips, radishes, and carrots. In salads, a good proportion is 70 percent pigmented vegetables to 30 percent greens.

Of course, this suggestion depends on the kind of activity a person engages in in his or her daily life. It is important to discharge as much energy as you are absorbing. If you engage in a great deal of physical and mental exertion as a matter of routine, there is little danger that you will consume more meat and/or pigmented vegetables than you burn up. On the other hand, a person who has achieved a very subtle state (which would be the only healthy reason for not engaging in a great deal of physical and mental exertion) is functioning on very fine energy and does not require meat or pigmented vegetables. Many people are very inactive both physically and creatively. The cure, of course, is to change one's routine; but until one has done so, there is not much sense in taking a lot of vitamins, which the body cannot store if it has no need of them. Nor is there any reason to eat large quantities of meat and pigmented vegetables; this additional energy will not be discharged, and it will only add to the organism's problem of stored-up, stagnating energy.

One brief note on the subject of vitamin supplements may be in order. Vitamin supplements will do you no good if you do not have sufficient trace elements in your body to activate them. It has been said that the urine of Americans is the most expensive urine in the world because it contains all the high-priced vitamins that are ingested and cannot be utilized. The elements and the cell salts are the inorganic bases that are minimally required if vitamins are to be effective. So, it is useless to take vitamins if you neglect the balance of minerals and trace elements. As we have seen, it may be necessary to take cell salts to adjust your mineral balance until the body can assimilate these important elements for itself.

## Fasting

Sudden fasting damages the body more than helps it. The body needs time to adjust to new eating habits, and therefore, the best way to fast is to take thirty-six days altogether: twelve days to build up to the fast, twelve days during which you do not take in anything but water, and twelve days to break the fast. During the first twelve days, there should be the following program of decreased food intake:

> 1st day: 3/4 breakfast + lunch + dinner
> 2d day: 1/2 breakfast + lunch + dinner
> 3d day: 1/4 breakfast + lunch + dinner
> 4th day: no breakfast + lunch + dinner
> 5th day: no breakfast + 3/4 lunch + dinner
> 6th day: no breakfast + 1/2 lunch + dinner
> 7th day: no breakfast + 1/4 lunch + dinner
> 8th day: no breakfast + no lunch + dinner
> 9th day: no breakfast + no lunch + 3/4 dinner
> 10th day: no breakfast + no lunch + 1/2 dinner
> 11th day: no breakfast + no lunch + 1/4 dinner
> 12th day: no food except water
>
> 12th day to 24th day: no food except water
> 25th day to 36th day: build back up to regular
> eating by starting to eat as on 11th day and
> reversing down to day 1, then resuming full meals.

## Taking Responsibility for Your Health

Our discussion of the processes of nutrition and assimilation has made it clear that how you live has a tremendous impact on your physical health. Health is not just the absence of disease; it is a dynamic, evolutionary process, a state of constant change. You are made up of some 350 trillion cells, each one unique and each with the capacity to maintain and reproduce itself and to interact and interrelate with all the other cells of the body. Every particle that makes up the components of the cell is in a state of constant activity, and there is a constant flow of energy arising from that activity. Because health is equivalent to the free, unimpeded flow of energy, you can see that it is possible to interfere with your health, to make yourself ill, by intervening on the subtlest, least material level.

The body is a wise organism. It will keep functioning if you do not interfere with it. Voluntary control really means allowing the body to control itself—by nonattachment, rather than by becoming attached to all the things that are going on in the body, by not thinking, rather than by thinking that you know better than the body.

Although, as we have seen, you are responsible for the state of your own health and also for your own healing, your mind by itself cannot sculpt out your own being. Your mind can only achieve its goals if the body is in a physiologically balanced state and an electromagnetically balanced condition. Mind and body are interdependent. So long as your body is not fully able to extract its energy needs autonomously from the outside, you will need to help it along by using cell salts, herbs, and a carefully adjusted diet. The immediate goal is to put the body back in balance so that you do not need to supplement it any longer. This will leave you free to focus on developing your mental and spiritual capacity, to follow the purposes indicated by your ray.

Your mind, like your body, will not attract the vibrations it needs for expansion unless it is already emitting those same vibrations that it hopes to attract. When you are able to do this, then, with your mind as a tool, you can do anything you want, as long as the mind is part of a healthy body to carry out its decisions fully.

Once you have begun to treat your physical problems with doses of the cell salts, which, in turn, will enable your body fluid to attract the elements it requires, then you must complement this process with a mental one. Just as you are expanding your body's ability to maintain its own balance, you must expand your mind and raise your overall energy level to emit subtler energy and thereby to attract more of it to yourself. As you lower the frequency and increase the amplitude of the vibrations of your physical being and so heighten the voltage of your ionically charged body fluid, you also automatically open up wider channels for expanded levels of consciousness. This is what we really mean when we talk about holistic medicine: a system of health maintenance that permits the free, unimpeded flow of energies, the expression of the potential of your whole self.

# 6 : The Tarot System of Natural Healing

In the preceding chapters of this book, we have discussed a number of approaches to health and the free expression of the abilities with which we were born. We have seen that such diverse approaches as meditation, the use of color and sound, herbs, nutrients, cell salts, and minerals can all help us to maintain the balance of physical, mental, and spiritual expression that we define as health.

For some years now, I have been working with a system that integrates these diverse forms of therapy and health maintenance by identifying for each person a symbol derived from the tarot deck that resonates with all the other health-maintaining influences he or she needs to use. The system is not infallible, and I am by no means satisfied that I have exhausted all the possibilities yet, but I have found that this tarot system will give me an accurate picture of an individual, even if he or she is not present. Later, when I actually see the person, the perceptions I have arrived at through the tarot system are generally confirmed, and many of the person's characteristics can be seen to fit together.

### The Origin of the Twenty-Two Cards of the Major Arcana

There is an anecdote in the arcane tradition that shortly before the capture of the ancient city of Alexandria and the burning of its famous Library, the high priests devised a way of preserving their esoteric knowledge. They analyzed their wisdom and derived twenty-two major mysteries and fifty-six minor mysteries. As a further security, these seventy-eight mysteries were translated into images that ultimately became the seventy-eight cards of the tarot deck.

The story goes that as these priests spread out across the world, they became nomads, gypsies, who preserved their ancient knowledge in the form of the mysteries of the tarot deck. And so the tradition developed of the gypsy fortune-teller who engaged in divination by the use of cards. The fifty-two cards of our common deck today are vestiges of the ancient tarot pack. The images have evolved from the original pictographs; going back only a few centuries, the symbols of the minor arcana (originally fifty-six cards) have changed from swords to spades, from wands to clubs, from cups to hearts, and from pentacles to diamonds.

Although the tarot deck is still used for fortune-telling today, its higher and more important purpose, according to tradition, was to preserve in symbolic form the laws of the universe as they were known to the ancient adepts. It is this symbolic value of the twenty-two cards of the major arcana of the tarot deck that we draw on in the tarot system of natural healing. As we shall see, the symbolism of a particular tarot card resonates with other forces and substances that are important to the person for whom that card represents his or her total essence.

We shall begin our introduction of the tarot system by describing the numerological procedures that are used to determine a person's tarot card.

## Name Number

The first component in determining your key numbers in the tarot system is the number derived from your name as it appears on your birth certificate. Your Name Number is determined by using your full name—first, middle, and family names—exactly as it was given to you at your birth. If "Jr." or "II" or "III" appeared on your birth certificate, this should be included as well, spelled out fully (Junior, Second, Third).

Even if you have never really used your full name as it appears on your birth certificate, or if you have stopped using it, it is this name that represents a matrix of energy, which was imprisoned within the imagery of your name and its numerological equivalent at the moment of your birth. You may feel that your name has very little to do with who you are, but it is possible that even before your birth, you may have had an influence on what name was given to you. While you were in your mother's womb, you were capable of telepathic communicating with your parents and may have played a part in deciding what name was selected for you.

Because the tarot system is based on Cabalistic numerology, you will need to use the Hebrew Cabalistic alphabet to find the number that corresponds to your name. The twenty-two characters of the Hebrew alphabet each have corresponding numbers; in translating this alphabet into its English equivalent, you will note that some numbers correspond to more than one letter and that some correspond to combinations of letters that represent single-letter consonants in the archaic Hebrew alphabet:

| | | |
|---|---|---|
| 1 = A | 9 = Th | 17 = F, Ph, P |
| 2 = B | 10 = I, J, Y | 18 = Sh, Ts, Tz |
| 3 = G | 11 = C, K | 19 = Q |
| 4 = D | 12 = L | 20 = R |
| 5 = E | 13 = M | 21 = S |
| 6 = U, V, W | 14 = N | 22 = T |
| 7 = Z | 15 = X | |
| 8 = H, Ch | 16 = O | |

Arrange your name in a vertical column—first, middle, and last names—and find the number equivalent for each letter (or combination of letters, when indicated above). The total of all the numbers corresponding to the letters in your name is your *Name Number*. For example, the name John Abel Peterson would look like this:

| | | | |
|---|---|---|---|
| J = 10 | A = 1 | P = 17 | 20 |
| O = 16 | B = 2 | E = 5 | 48 |
| H = 8 | E = 5 | T = 22 | +120 |
| N = 14 | L = 12 | E = 5 | 188 = Name Number |
| 48 | 20 | E = 5 | |
| | | R = 20 | |
| | | S = 21 | |
| | | O = 16 | |
| | | N = 14 | |
| | | 120 | |

## Birth Number

Next, find your *Birth Number* by writing the numbers corresponding to your birth date in a vertical column. If John Abel Peterson was born on September 7, 1931 (or 9/7/1931), his Birth Number would look like this:

$$9$$
$$7$$
$$1$$
$$9$$
$$3$$
$$\underline{1}$$
$$30 = \textit{Birth Number}$$

## Soul Number and Soul Essence

The first essential quality derived in the tarot system is the *Soul Number,* which is then translated into the Soul Essence. To determine the Soul Number, add the Birth Number and the Name Number. Using the same example, the Soul Number for John Abel Peterson would be:

$$188$$
$$\underline{+30}$$
$$218 = \text{Soul Number}$$

In determining the Soul Essence (and also the Mental Essence, Physical Essence, and Diagnostic Number below), any number above 22 must be reduced because there are only 22 tarot cards used in the system. Thus, using our example:

$$\text{Soul Number} = 218$$
$$\text{Soul Essence} = 2 + 1 + 8 = 11$$

As you will see when you refer to pages 116 and 134, tarot card no. 11 is Justice; so, the Soul Essence of John Abel Peterson is represented by the symbolism of Justice.

The Soul Essence is the power, the energy with which you are born into the world. It reflects your purpose in life, the function of your soul. This essence exists whether you manifest it or not; it is your toolbox, the potential that is reflected in your ray.

If, after adding the digits of the Soul Number together, you still get a number over 22, add the digits of the new number together, until you get a number under 23.

If the Soul Number has a zero in it, then the digits are added and the zero is thrown out. For example, Soul Number 103 reduces to 4 (1 + 0 + 3), not 13 (10 + 3). But if the Soul Number is 148, then the Soul Essence will be 1 + 4 + 8 = 13.

## Mental Essence

Next we derive the Mental Essence. Subtract the Soul Essence from the Soul Number, then divide by 9 (because everything is in cycles of 9 in the tarot system):

$$\frac{\text{Soul Number} - \text{Soul Essence}}{9} = \frac{218 - 11}{9} = \frac{207}{9} = 23 \qquad 9$$

(The resulting number should always be a whole number. If you get a fraction, you made an error in your arithmetic.)

Because 23 is above 22, reduce by adding the digits:

$$2 + 3 = 5 = \text{Mental Essence}$$

The Mental Essence is the directing force of your mind and will. In this case, it is expressed by card no. 5, the Hierophant (see pages 126–127).

## Physical Essence

The symbolic number for Physical Essence is obtained by adding the constant 1 (for one expressive act) to the Mental Essence. In our example,

$$\text{Mental Essence} + 1 = \text{Physical Essence}$$
$$5 + 1 = 6 = \text{Physical Essence}$$

The Physical Essence number refers to the actual expression you give to your energy; obviously, this may differ from the expression proposed by your mind and will. In our example, the Physical Essence is represented by no. 6, the Lovers.

## Total Essence or Diagnostic Number

Your Total Essence is obtained by adding together the symbolic numbers of the Soul, the Mind, and the Body:

| | |
|---|---|
| Soul Essence | 11 |
| Mental Essence | 5 |
| Physical Essence | 6 |
| | 22 = Total Essence or Diagnostic Number |

In our example, then, the Diagnostic Number is represented by no. 22, the Fool. All the therapeutics connected with the Fool in the discussion that follows would serve as preventive guidelines for John Abel Peterson.

Because one aspect of your being—soul, mind, or body—may be more developed or active than the others, it does no harm to keep in mind the corresponding tarot card for each element. However, the discussion of the individual tarot cards in this chapter refers only to the card for the Total Essence, or Diagnostic Number, for each individual.

## Variations

In addition to determining the card that represents your Total Essence, based on your Soul Essence, Mental Essence, and Physical Essence, you can derive further insight into the influences of each day by determining your Daily Total Essence. Suppose today's date is October 14, 1979 (10/14/1979). Derive a Date Number as you did for your Birth Number:

$$
\begin{array}{l}
1 \\
0 \\
1 \\
4 \\
1 \\
9 \\
7 \\
\underline{9} \\
32 = \text{Date Number}
\end{array}
$$

Add this new Date Number to your Diagnostic Number (22 in our example):

$$32 + 22 = 54$$

Because this is over 23, we add the digits:

$$5 + 4 = 9 = \text{new Diagnostic Number for 10/14/1979}$$

Thus, for October 14, 1979, John Abel Peterson may use card no. 9, the Hermit, as his diagnostic card if he wishes. For people whose diagnostic cards are very broad in their application—no. 10, the Wheel of Fortune, for example—it can be particularly helpful to work with a new Diagnostic Number for a specific day.

Some people go through a distinct rebirth during the course of their lives, sometimes even more than one. Although you keep the same Name Number throughout your life, you would determine a new Birth Number (and hence a new Soul Essence, Mental Essence, Physical

Essence, and Total Essence, or Diagnostic Number) by taking the date on which you experienced your rebirth as your new birthdate.

Such rebirths are not uncommon. In my counseling work, I sometimes see an individual in whose energy fields I observe a growth pattern that indicates that they have gone through a drastic stage in which they transcended everything they had previously been expressing in their lives. They can then be given a new Birth Number corresponding to the date on which that graduation day took place, and an astrologer can make a new natal chart based on that new date as well as the time and place where the graduation occurred. Such new Birth Numbers and natal charts will reflect the drastic changes that have taken place in these people's lives, the new set of tools they are now working with.

## The Twenty-Two Cards of the Major Arcana

The Total Essence Number, or Diagnostic Number, that you have determined by the procedure just described above refers to the corresponding tarot card. Because there are only twenty-two cards, the number must be 22 or less. The twenty-two cards are listed below, with their symbolic meanings:

| 1 | Magician | Truth |
|---|---|---|
| 2 | High Priestess | Wisdom |
| 3 | Empress | Authority on love |
| 4 | Emperor | Authority on world process |
| 5 | Hierophant | Authority on magic |
| 6 | Lovers | Communication, discrimination |
| 7 | Chariot | Triumph, victory |
| 8 | Strength | Art, control |
| 9 | Hermit | Illumination |
| 10 | Wheel of Fortune | Worldly process |
| 11 | Justice | Balance of vital powers |
| 12 | Hanged Man | Transition |
| 13 | Death | Regeneration |
| 14 | Temperance | Symbolical language |
| 15 | Devil | Removal of opacity |
| 16 | Tower | Removal of physical obstacles |
| 17 | Star | Supernal powers |
| 18 | Moon | Reflection |
| 19 | Sun | Renewal |
| 20 | Judgment | Awakening |

| 21 | World | Change |
| 22 | Fool | All-encompassing light |

These twenty-two cards are symbolic of all the laws operating in our lives. As symbols, they are not the truth in themselves; rather, they are intended to guide the mind toward the attainment of truth. Remember that this system is merely a tool; the ultimate objective is to express the energy that we are, our Soul Essence.

I have found that the tarot cards also have a relationship to the symbolism of astrological signs and planets and to astronomical situations in our galaxy. The cards also are associated with different colors. We have already seen that each color has a certain frequency, or vibrational rate, and that these frequencies also correspond to musical notes. All these relationships, then, are built up through what I call *comparative affinities;* because they all resonate to the same frequency, they are all interrelated.

I have noted elsewhere in this book that like attracts like in the paramagnetic fields of the human body. Thus, when you are vibrating on a certain frequency, you tend to attract those particles that you need that are also associated with the same frequency. Similarly, certain plants need to be under a specific astrological influence, in a certain color light (i.e., to resonate on a certain frequency) in order to grow to fruition. Minerals, too, are associated with different frequencies. Thus, using the concept of comparative affinities, I have indicated for each card the curative agents and health-maintaining substances that will be most effective for people who resonate on the same frequency as that card.

Disease and malfunction are symptoms that the mind and body are not in harmony with the Soul Essence. The cards provide a means of synthesizing all three of these elements into a coherent regimen of health and well-being. Knowledge of your card will help you to take proper preventive measures. Every person needs a balanced diet with appropriate vitamins and minerals. But there will be a tendency for each person to have more problems with particular body functions because of his or her role in the universe. It is this specific role that the cards help to identify. The diseases mentioned are those to which you will be most susceptible because of your resonance with a certain frequency; they are not the diseases that you will necessarily get. Disease is the consequence of improperly using or making no use of one's energies, of holding back and resisting expression. This is usually due to external influences to which we are subjected, which make it difficult to live in a state of nonattachment. Moreover, you cannot express your function in life if your body is not healthy.

The health of the mind is equally urgent; like the body, the mind functions best when it is fully involved in life but at the same time nonattached. Neither the body nor the mind can infallibly help the other. It is our Soul Essence, our innate deposit of energy, that can effect the unification of these three elements; it is as intuition that our Soul Essence, which is stable, directs the mind, and it is the mind that directs the body.

In order to stimulate our Soul Essence, we can use particular colors and sounds that can help to activate our intuition about ourselves, bring it out and express it.

Not surprisingly, total enlightenment means no color, no sounds, and no influences. A person in a state of total enlightenment, or Christ consciousness, functions surrounded by white light, not by the hues determined by the various states of our seven energy centers, or chakras. As *Voluntary Controls* tried to make clear, spiritual growth is marked by the increasing brightening of our auras, the increasing nonattachment from external influences. I think that every human being has the potential for reaching this state of enlightenment.

With these thoughts in mind, let us now examine each card and its associated regimen of health. The discussion of each card is divided into four sections:

*A:* The astrological affinities of the card, along with the color, sound, and frequency with which the symbolism of the card resonates. Previous chapters in this book have already made you aware that there are colors and musical notes associated with each of the body's energy centers and assimilative processes.

*B:* General themes for personal development. Soul expression refers to the tools we are given at birth for the accomplishment of our potentialities. The human expression suggests the manner in which we need to carry out our potentials in daily life.

*C:* Common disorders for each character type, with appropriate therapies, including herbal remedies for each ailment. (See Chapter 5 and Appendix A for further discussions of how to use herbs.)

*D:* General ingredients for health maintenance. The items included for each card are selected largely according to their astrological affinity to the particular card; they do not represent a medically recommended regimen for the person represented by that card. You should familiarize yourself with all the herbs, vitamins, cell salts, minerals, and trace elements if you are going to undertake thorough self-analysis and healing. This book provides you with a basic approach to several classes of these healing agents.

Once you have determined which tarot card corresponds to your

Diagnostic Number, you can assess whether the affinities for your card seem to ring true.

## Tarot Astrology

Twelve of the twenty-two tarot cards are associated with a zodiac sign as well as with a planet; the remaining ten cards have planetary influences only. People with diagnostic cards among the ten without zodiac signs are influenced by all the signs of the zodiac in a fluctuating manner. We might compare this difference with hearing and being influenced by only one string of a stringed instrument, as opposed to being affected by all the strings at once. In the first case, we resonate

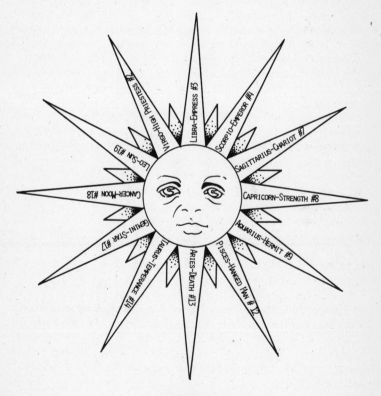

**FIGURE 12:**

**CARDS WITH ZODIAC SIGNS**

with a single frequency; and in the latter, with all frequencies. People whose diagnostic card is not associated with a zodiac sign often find it useful to gain further information by determining the Diagnostic Number for the particular date in question, which is done by deriving a new Date Number and adding it to the Diagnostic Number, as outlined on pages 115–116.

The cards that have zodiac signs are shown in Figure 12. The signs, with their corresponding tarot cards, are in the customary sequence around the wheel of the zodiac. This means that each card will be influenced by its *aspects,* or angles, with other zodiac signs.

In tarot astrology, when a card and a sign are *opposing,* they are at an 180-degree angle; thus, the sign opposing card no. 2 (High Priestess) is Pisces (see Figure 12). When two influences are *squaring,* they are at a 90-degree angle; thus, for each card, two squarings are possible. For no. 2, the High Priestess, the squares are with Gemini and Sagittarius.

Planets are the other source of astrological influences for the tarot cards in this system. Table 5 shows these planetary influences for the twenty-two cards.

### TABLE 5: PLANETS FOR THE TAROT CARDS

| Cards without Zodiac Signs | Planets | Cards with Zodiac Signs |
|---|---|---|
| no. 1 Magician | Mercury | |
| | Mercury | no. 2 High Priestess |
| | Venus | no. 3 Empress |
| | Pluto | no. 4 Emperor |
| no. 5 Hierophant | Jupiter | |
| no. 6 Lovers | Venus | |
| | Jupiter | no. 7 Chariot |
| | Saturn | no. 8 Strength |
| | Uranus | no. 9 Hermit |
| no. 10 Wheel of Fortune | All planets | |
| no. 11 Justice | Neptune | |
| | Neptune | no. 12 Hanged Man |
| | Mars | no. 13 Death |
| | Venus | no. 14 Temperance |
| no. 15 Devil | Saturn | |
| no. 16 Tower | Mars | |
| | Mercury | no. 17 Star |
| | Moon | no. 18 Moon |
| | Sun | no. 19 Sun |
| no. 20 Judgment | Moon | |
| no. 21 World | Sun | |
| no. 22 Fool | All planets | |

## The Tarot Cards

### no. 1 *The Magician*

A. *Characteristics*
1. TOTAL ESSENCE: truth and dexterity; using dexterity to put truth into practice.
2. ZODIAC SIGN: none
3. PLANET: Mercury
4. COLOR: violet
5. MUSICAL NOTE: B
6. FREQUENCY: 493.9 cps

B. *Themes for Personal Development*
1. SOUL EXPRESSION: utilization of all the energies and forces found within the cosmic system for the implementation of truth.
2. HUMAN EXPRESSION: spiritual leadership that is not yet apparent.

C. *Common Disorders*
1. GENERAL AILMENTS: nervous and respiratory disorders.
2. THERAPY: need for all kinds of therapies, not just herbal remedies: reveries, meditation, massage, hypnosis, psychosynthesis, natural therapies—anything that enables persons falling into this card to become more aware of truth and their role in implementing it.

D. *Health Maintenance*
1. HERBS: celery / cumin seeds and fruit / devil's bit / elecampane / fennel seeds / hazelnut / lavender / licorice / lily of the valley / *mandrake root / mulberry / myrtle / parsley / parsnip / sedges / sweet marjoram / valerian / wood sage
2. VITAMINS: B complex
3. CELL SALTS: potassium chloride (KALI-MUR)
4. MINERALS: Mercury
5. DIETARY NEEDS: almonds / beef liver / carrot greens and root / cucumbers / egg yolk / endive / green leaf vegetables / herring / lettuce / lima beans / mackerel / parsley / parsnip greens and root / seeds (all) / tuna / wheat grass
6. ELEMENTS AND/OR TRACE ELEMENTS: actinium: spleen stimulant / cobalt: cardiac depressant / gallium: depressant for lymphatic system / radon: motor depressant, builder of leucocytes

## no. 2 *The High Priestess*

A. *Characteristics*
1. TOTAL ESSENCE: wisdom, the utmost of knowing; the moon, reflection of truth, which removes the shrouds of ignorance through diligent searching.
2. ZODIAC SIGN: Virgo
3. PLANET: Mercury
4. COLOR: dark violet
5. MUSICAL NOTE: low B
6. FREQUENCY: 466.1 cps

B. *Themes for Personal Development*
1. SOUL EXPRESSION: awareness of absolute beingness; consciousness of one's own holistic beingness, circumscribing the past, present, and future in a reflection of union and total perception of both the visible and the invisible in the now.
2. HUMAN EXPRESSION: the implications of mental perception and the comprehension thereof; intuitive insight applied; inspiration; the union of all polarities, achieved through synchronization of the two hemispheres of the brain.

C. *Common Disorders*
1. GENERAL AILMENTS: intestinal disturbances
   a. Gas, colitis, colic, and so on: caraway seed / cumin seed / gingerroot / goldenseal / peppermint / psyllium seed / *wormwood (also used for moxibustion, pyramids of wormwood placed on affected spot and burned)
   b. Malnutrition, stemming from poor protein digestion: American centaury root / dandelion root / Irish moss / sorrel / strawberry leaves / yogurt (to build up intestinal flora)
2. INFLUENCES ON VIRGO:
   a. Squaring with Sagittarius:
   For activation and regulation of the liver: cleavers / Oregon graperoot
   For rheumatism: black cohosh / cod-liver oil (daily) / sarsaparilla / Stay away from citrus fruit and citrus-based soft drinks. Have copper level checked; arthritis is tied to copper deficiency. Have glucose tolerance test for hypoglycemia.
   b. Opposing to Pisces:
   For mucous discharge: comfrey root / marshmallow root / mullein

    c. Squaring with Gemini:
       For weakness of the chest, pulmonary conditions: hyssop /
       pleurisy root / ribwort
       For nervousness: hops / oats / passionflower / wood betony

D. *Health Maintenance*
  1. HERBS: horehound / marjoram (may also be mixed with oil for
    a liniment) / mulberry / scullcap / wild sage / *woodbine /
    For activation of gastric glands to assure better protein
    digestion, bromelin (pineapple enzyme) is used, often
    combined with papain (pineapple enzyme).
  2. VITAMINS: total B complex, especially $B_{15}$ (pangamic acid)
  3. CELL SALTS: potassium sulfate (KALI-SULPH): sulfur for cleaning
    and potassium for nerve activation.
  4. MINERALS: zinc
  5. DIETARY NEEDS: almonds / apricots / barley / chicory /
    endive / oats / rye / protein foods in general
  6. ELEMENTS AND/OR TRACE ELEMENTS: chromium: cerebral
    depressant / fluorine: acute alterative / nickel: a tonic /
    niobium: a skin builder / zinc: antipruritic (anti-itching); good
    for nervous headaches and neuralgia and for stimulation of the
    senses; also aids against phlebitis and as a curative for diabetes.

## no. 3 *The Empress*

A. *Characteristics*
  1. TOTAL ESSENCE: the authority on love in its totality.
  2. ZODIAC SIGN: Libra
  3. PLANET: Venus
  4. COLOR: light yellow
  5. MUSICAL NOTE: high E
  6. FREQUENCY: 659.3 cps

B. *Themes for Personal Development*
  1. SOUL EXPRESSION: supreme power balanced by active intelli-
    gence and transformed into wisdom; the balance and germina-
    tion of love by action.
  2. HUMAN EXPRESSION: union by knowing and enlightenment. If
    one is enlightened, he or she knows. If one knows, he or she
    becomes enlightened. Knowledge is based on the authority of
    another, as opposed to knowingness, which is based on an author-
    ity beyond and within one; on intuition. To go from knowledge to
    knowingness is to transmute intellect into wisdom. Love is the
    essence of such knowingness, based on trust of the inner authority.

C. *Common Disorders*

   1. GENERAL AILMENTS:

     a. Kidney problems (stemming from holding back feelings), crystallization (because of overintellectualization): buchu leaves / corn silk / juniper berries / parsley root / wild carrot

     b. Diabetes: huckleberry / Check for insulin and zinc deficiency.

     c. Weak eyes: cucumber slices applied to eyelids / eyebright / fennel

     d. Rheumatic fever: huckleberry (drink 3 times daily) / Check for zinc deficiency.

     e. Lumbago: blueberry leaves / damiana / goldenrod / heartsease / Jerusalem artichoke leaves / pansy / sarsaparilla

     f. Intestinal pressure, gas: activated charcoal capsules

   2. INFLUENCES ON LIBRA:

     a. Squaring with Capricorn:
     Teeth and bone care: carrageen / plantain / restharrow / shave grass / silica
     Skin troubles: chickweed / comfrey / shepherd's purse / yellow dock

     b. Opposing to Aries:
     Head colds and headaches: boneset / comfrey / elecampane / sage / senega root
     Nervous disorders, insomnia: chamomile / linden flowers / CALMS tablets (a combination of cell salts) and CALMS Forte (a combination of cell salts with herbs such as valerian, passionflower, hops, oats).
     Mucous discharges and restlessness: wood betony

     c. Squaring with Cancer:
     Aging and aching of the muscular system: shave grass (contains silica) / silica cell salts
     Gastric distress: aniseed / cinnamon bark / gingerroot / peppermint / thyme

D. *Health Maintenance*

   1. HERBS: balm / knotgrass / lemon leaves and fruit / pansy / primrose / strawberry leaves, tops, and stems / violet / watercress / white rose / wild thyme

   2. VITAMINS: A and E

3. CELL SALTS: sodium phosphate (NATRUM-PHOS) (especially for kidney and intestinal problems)
4. MINERALS: manganese, especially for pituitary gland
5. DIETARY NEEDS: bran / brown rice / citrus fruits / eggs / figs / fish and fish oils / green leaf vegetables
6. ELEMENTS AND/OR TRACE ELEMENTS: argon: arterial stimulant / dysprosium: energizes kidney and gallbladder / erbium: genital excitant / holmium: aphrodisiac / lutetium: emmenagogue / manganese: vasoconstrictor / thallium: ecbolic (promotes labor) / ytterbium: sex builder, for the gonads / (All these can be found in kelp, dulse, red beets.)

## no. 4 The Emperor

A. *Characteristics*

1. TOTAL ESSENCE: ruler of the physical world; authority and example of the worldly process.
2. ZODIAC SIGN: Scorpio
3. PLANET: Pluto
4. COLOR: dark red
5. MUSICAL NOTE: low C
6. FREQUENCY: 261.6 cps

B. *Themes for Personal Development*

1. SOUL EXPRESSION: realization of perpetual forces and their position of authority in the worldly process.
2. HUMAN EXPRESSION: absorption of electromagnetic forces; the person with that card is to be both the receiver and the transmitter, instantaneously, without a lag between the two functions.

C. *Common Disorders*

1. GENERAL AILMENTS:
   a. Poor elimination (arising from failure to perform the receiving and transmitting functions without lag): agar-agar / *blue flag root / buckthorn root / butternut bark / psyllium seeds / *rhubarb root
   b. Bladder disorders: corn silk / parsley root / wild carrot greens
   c. Inflammation of the genitals, colon, bladder, kidneys: slippery elm
2. INFLUENCES ON SCORPIO:
   a. Squaring with Aquarius:

For problems with blood circulation: burdock root / elder
root / gentian root / red raspberry leaves

b. Opposing to Taurus:
For throat problems: honey / horehound / licorice root /
quince seeds / wild cherry bark (use with slippery elm bark
lozenges)

c. Squaring with Leo:
For nervous tension: chamomile / coriander seeds / hops /
linden flowers / oats / passionflower / pimpernel / sweet
basil / valerian root

D. *Health Maintenance*
1. HERBS: blackthorn root and berries / bramble / horehound /
*wormwood (use as external poultice with water)
2. VITAMINS: B complex, especially $B_{12}$ (for stress), C, and E; $B_6$
(for cerebral and spinal problems, no more than 100 to 150
milligrams daily)
3. CELL SALTS: Calcium sulfate (CALC-SULPH), for metabolism
4. MINERALS: Iron
5. DIETARY NEEDS: asparagus / beets / black cherries / prunes /
radishes / soybean products / wheat germ
6. ELEMENTS AND/OR TRACE ELEMENTS: cadmium: stimulant of
sensory system / hydrogen: liver energizer / krypton and
neon: irritants, but good for building red blood cells

## no. 5 The Hierophant (The Pope or High Priest)

A. *Characteristics*
1. TOTAL ESSENCE: The authority on magic; the holy father, cause
of the wholeness of things, implementing in the physical world
the truth of the Magician (Card number 1), bringing higher teach-
ings down to practical levels.
2. ZODIAC SIGN: none
3. PLANET: Jupiter
4. COLOR: royal blue, ultramarine
5. MUSICAL NOTE: G
6. FREQUENCY: 392 cps

B. *Themes for Personal Development*
1. SOUL EXPRESSION: universal law; the regulation of the infinite
being in unity, the unity of all substances; alchemical integration
of the opposing forces in all substances.
2. HUMAN EXPRESSION: communication by vibrations and reso-

nance; the trial of an individual by freedom and action; knowledge makes us free, and freedom is expressed by spontaneity and inspiration.

C. *Common Disorders*

  1. GENERAL AILMENTS: blood disorders and malnutrition.
  2. THERAPY: proper diet; electromagnetic therapy: radionics, radiesthesia, acupuncture, auric healing, magnetic healing, polarity, and pyramid therapy.

D. *Health Maintenance*

  1. HERBS: agrimony / common oak / fig / houseleek / jasmine / maple / olive / thistle / water avens / wood betony
  2. VITAMINS: practically all
  3. CELL SALTS: See Note. Especially iron phosphate (FER-PHOS).
  4. MINERALS: tin. See Note.
  5. DIETARY NEEDS: copper- and iron-containing foods / copper: apricot kernels, legumes, nuts, whole grains / iron: dulse, kelp, green leafy vegetables, liver, sesame seed, squash seed
     See Note.
  6. ELEMENTS AND/OR TRACE ELEMENTS: See Note.

## no. 6 The Lovers

A. *Characteristics*

  1. TOTAL ESSENCE: the balance of male and female, positive and negative; Integration of the polarity of life as we know it, as a constant current that unites the two poles.
  2. ZODIAC SIGN: none
  3. PLANET: Venus
  4. COLOR: canary yellow
  5. MUSICAL NOTE: E
  6. FREQUENCY: 329.6 cps

B. *Themes for Personal Development*

  1. SOUL EXPRESSION: the balance of positive and negative, of liberty and necessity; freedom through recognition of both male and female aspects in us.
  2. HUMAN EXPRESSION: to be responsible for every insight and emotion, to nourish them and bring them to form and expression.

Note: For dietary needs, cell salts, minerals, and trace elements, choices should be determined by the ailments occurring in the person with this diagnostic card. Also, for further guidance, calculate the new Diagnostic Number for the specific date (see pages 115–116).

## C. *Common Disorders*

1. GENERAL AILMENTS: disorders of the renal system; fluid retention.

2. THERAPY: all diuretics; rest and recreation; time for persons on this card to recuperate by themselves to bring out their creativity. Their fluid retention is caused mainly by their emotionalism.

## D. *Health Maintenance*

1. HERBS: bay leaves / birch shoots and leaves / blackberry / elder / fleabane / kidney bean / lady's bedstraw / orchids / oxeye daisy / peach / *pennyroyal seeds and root / peppermint / scavius / spearmint / *tansy / wild apple

2. VITAMINS: See Note.

3. CELL SALTS: See Note.

4. MINERALS: copper

5. DIETARY NEEDS: See Note.

6. ELEMENTS AND/OR TRACE ELEMENTS: argon: arterial stimulant / dysprosium: renal energizer / erbium: genital excitant / holmium: aphrodisiac / lutetium: emmenagogue / manganese: vasoconstrictor / thallium: ecbolic (promotes labor) / ytterbium: sex builder

## *no. 7 The Chariot*

### A. *Characteristics*

1. TOTAL ESSENCE: riding on the four elements, the chariot is the earth, pulled by the black and white sphinxes, representing the union of positive and negative. The charioteer does not need to hold the reins, for he is led by inner truth; he has triumphed over the dual aspects within himself and has become whole.

2. ZODIAC SIGN: Sagittarius

3. PLANET: Jupiter

4. COLOR: light purple

5. MUSICAL NOTE: high A

6. FREQUENCY: 466.1 cps

### B. *Themes for Personal Development*

1. SOUL EXPRESSION: union of spirit (energy) and matter; the submission of the elements and forces of the cosmos through control

Note: This is one of the cards that is not associated with a specific zodiac sign. For further guidance in health maintenance, determine the new Diagnostic Number for the specific date in question (see pages 115–116).

of energy (spirit) over mind, of mind over matter, through nonattachment combined with full involvement.

2. HUMAN EXPRESSION: dominion over the elements; supervision. To overcome being dominated by any force, seek a higher goal for energy. In exercising dominion, the goal is nonattachment; flowing, benevolent control of one's subjects.

## C. *Common Disorders*

1. GENERAL AILMENTS:
   a. Arthritis and rheumatism (arising from power tending to make these individuals rigid): black cohosh / celery seeds / cod-liver oil / knotgrass / sarsaparilla / wahoo
   b. Liver ailments: cleavers / dandelion root / liverwort / Oregon graperoot
   c. Obesity: burdock root / elder root / pokeroot
      Plus creative work to counteract boredom, which leads to overeating.

2. INFLUENCES ON SAGITTARIUS:
   a. Squaring with Pisces:
      For colds and mucous discharge: coltsfoot / comfrey root / elecampane / gum arabic / maidenhair fern
   b. Opposing to Gemini:
      For chest weakness: bloodroot / hyssop / pleurisy root / ribwort
   c. Squaring with Virgo:
      For digestive tract problems: cumin seeds / ginger / goldenseal / peppermint / *wormwood
      For nervousness: catnip / valerian / yellow lady's-slipper

## D. *Health Maintenance*

1. HERBS: agrimony (with yarrow and slippery elm, a good tea for varicose veins) / asparagus / balm / bloodwort / borage / couch grass / dandelion / feverfew / figs / huckleberry / hyssop / leeks / marshmallow root / sage / sugarcane / wood betony / yellow dock
2. VITAMINS: C and E
3. CELL SALTS: silicea
4. MINERALS: tin
5. DIETARY NEEDS: carrot greens / liver / oats / parsnips / rice and rice bran / cucumbers, melons, and squashes (for their silicea content)
6. ELEMENTS AND/OR TRACE ELEMENTS: bromine: stimulant for venous system / europium: depressant for renal system /

gadolinium: antimalarial / ytterbium: vasodilator, hypnotic, narcotic, antipyretic, analgesic, anaphrodisiac, sex builder

## no. 8 Strength (or Art)

### A. *Characteristics*

1. TOTAL ESSENCE: creativity, derived from mastery of one's animalistic nature through the proper use of the energies involved, through the development of self-discipline. Creativity is, then, following one's intuition.
2. ZODIAC SIGN: Capricorn
3. PLANET: Saturn
4. COLOR: dark blue
5. MUSICAL NOTE: low G
6. FREQUENCY: 370.1 cps

### B. *Themes for Personal Development*

1. SOUL EXPRESSION: finding the balance between attraction and repulsion.
2. HUMAN EXPRESSION: to temper one's expression and receptivity in order to grow aware of the inner authority; quieting of outward activity in order to hear the inner voice.

### C. *Common Disorders*

1. GENERAL AILMENTS:
   a. Hypoglycemia (low blood sugar): Mostly dietary approach: high-protein diet, dairy products, fish, fowl, soybeans, low salt intake. Fruits, especially: apricots, figs, dates, persimmons. Vegetables, especially spinach, endive, beans, lettuce. Foods high in copper content: soybeans, lettuce, all beans and all seeds (copper activates glycogen in the liver). Tomatoes, cayenne pepper, apricot kernels.
   b. Arthritis and rheumatism: black cohosh / celery seed / columbo root / dulse / kelp / knotgrass / Peruvian bark / sarsaparilla / sassafras
   c. Skin disorders: chickweed / marjoram / shepherd's purse / yellow dock
   d. Problems with nails, skeleton, teeth: meadowsweet flowers / nettles / restharrow / shave grass / sweet flag
   e. For nerves: bloodroot / hops / valerian / CALMS (see no. 14, Empress) / passionflower
2. INFLUENCES ON CAPRICORN:
   a. Squaring with Aries:

For head colds: American pennyroyal / blue vervain / boneset / coltsfoot / comfrey root / rosemary / turtlebloom / sages

b. Opposing to Cancer:

For digestive tract problems: aniseseed / bitterwood / caraway seeds / cinnamon bark / cumin seeds / flaxseed / gingerroot / peppermint / woodruff

c. Squaring with Libra:

For kidney disorders (especially sluggish kidneys): corn silk / goldenrod / juniper berries / kidneywort / parsley root / upland cranberry / wild carrot

D. *Health Maintenance*

1. HERBS: *belladonna / *blue flag root / buckthorn / *henbane leaves / mullein leaves (boil in milk) / shepherd's purse / Solomon's seal

2. VITAMINS: A, C, and E

3. CELL SALTS: calcium phosphate (CALC-PHOS) (calcium for tissue insulation, phosphate for calcium and magnesium metabolism and as a nutrient for the thyroid and pituitary glands)

4. MINERALS: lead

5. DIETARY NEEDS: acerola cherries / barley / bran / broccoli / brown rice / carrots / citrus fruits / cod-liver oil / eggs / lentils / parsley / red peppers / rose hips / rye / spinach / yams / yogurt

6. ELEMENTS AND/OR TRACE ELEMENTS: cesium: antipruritic / indium: diaphoretic / oxygen: anodyne, demulcent, febrifuge, vitality builder

## no. 9 *The Hermit*

A. *Characteristics*

1. TOTAL ESSENCE: illumination. The hooded, black-robed figure holding a lantern with a six-pointed star shows the integration of the above and the below; an important symbol for the Age of Aquarius.

2. ZODIAC SIGN: Aquarius

3. PLANET: Uranus

4. COLOR: light blue

5. MUSICAL NOTE: high G

6. FREQUENCY: 415.5 cps

B. *Themes for Personal Development*
1. SOUL EXPRESSION: absolute wisdom, the result of total illumination.
2. HUMAN EXPRESSION: directing of will power, circumspection, and guiding all actions by recognition of divine will. "Not my will, but Thy will" is the test of proper guidance, which comes from intuitive sources, rather than from conscious thought processes.

C. *Common Disorders*
1. GENERAL AILMENTS:
   a. Stagnant blood circulation (headache, poor circulation), arising from failure to follow intuitive forces: gentian root / red raspberry leaves / sweet basil
   b. To condition the blood: alfalfa / bladder wrack / dulse / nettles / sassafras bark / spikenard
   c. Cramps and spasms, arising from improper calcium metabolism: shave grass / silicea / sunflower seeds
   d. Nervousness: chamomile / scullcap / wood betony / yellow lady's-slipper
   e. External skin care: heal-all / Saint-John's-wort / sweet fern / witch hazel
2. INFLUENCES ON AQUARIUS:
   a. Squaring with Taurus:
   For throat afflictions: arrowroot / flaxseed / honey / licorice root / marshmallow root / slippery elm
   b. Opposing to Leo:
   For heart disorders: cayenne pepper / coriander seeds / culver's root / sweet basil / *wild geranium root
   For blood purification: cayenne pepper / red raspberry leaves
   c. Squaring with Scorpio:
   For bladder disorders: corn silk / wild carrot greens
   For poor elimination: buckthorn / psyllium seeds / *rhubarb root

D. *Health Maintenance*
1. HERBS: apricots / cinquefoil / couch grass / dandelion / myrrh / red rose / sassafras (use like cucumbers for eyewash) / spikenard / *tansy / thistle
2. VITAMINS: C and E
3. CELL SALTS: sodium chloride (NATRUM-MUR)
4. MINERALS: Lodestone (found in roots, volcanic ash)
5. DIETARY NEEDS: acerola cherries / apples / Brazil nuts / brewers' yeast / cheese (hard) / eggs / honey / lemons / pecans / turnip greens / walnuts

6. ELEMENTS AND/OR TRACE ELEMENTS: carbon: for the eliminative trace, a motor stimulant / manganese: nutrient for pituitary gland / molybdenum: tonic / palladium: lymph activator / platinum: depressant for the spleen / rhodium: digestant / ruthenium: cathartic / sodium: cholagogue, balancer and stabilizer / tin: nerve builder / tungsten: nerve builder

## no. 10 The Wheel of Fortune

A. *Characteristics*
  1. TOTAL ESSENCE: The axis, with all the human and cosmic powers and aspects synthesized, the worldly process in its totality.
  2. ZODIAC SIGN: all
  3. PLANET: all
  4. COLOR: white, which includes and reflects all colors, iridescent white.
  5. MUSICAL: the sounds of the total musical scale, such as chimes.
  6. FREQUENCY: none

B. *Themes for Personal Development*
No specific themes. See Note.

C. *Common Disorders*
  1. GENERAL AILMENTS: The person with this card is constantly fluctuating because he or she is subject to all the influences represented by the other cards. See Note.
  2. THERAPY: All therapies in their natural form: physiotherapy, hydrotherapy, herbology, biochemicals, and so on; subtle electric therapies, such as ultrasound, infrared, ultraviolet, diathermy.

D. *Health Maintenance*
  1. HERBS: See Note.
  2. VITAMINS: See Note.
  3. CELL SALTS: See Note.
  4. MINERALS: See Note.
  5. DIETARY NEEDS: See Note.
  6. ELEMENTS AND/OR TRACE ELEMENTS: See Note.

Note: Because people on this card are constantly fluctuating, they should have access to all forms of therapy and all remedies; virtually any therapy could work for them. For additional guidance, determine the Diagnostic Number for the particular day in question by adding the original Diagnostic Number, 10, to the new Date Number.

### no. 11 Justice

A. *Characteristics*
   1. TOTAL ESSENCE: balance of vital powers, of night and day, sun and moon; impartial, seeking within rather than being influenced by outer appearances; a master card.
   2. ZODIAC SIGN: none
   3. PLANET: Neptune
   4. COLOR: white (iridescent)
   5. MUSICAL NOTE: music of the spheres
   6. FREQUENCY: none

B. *Themes for Personal Development*
   1. SOUL EXPRESSION: the expression of dualistic forces, of the spiritual and the material.
   2. HUMAN EXPRESSION: the application of balanced perception and transmission.

C. *Common Disorders*
   1. GENERAL AILMENTS: Kidney disorders, urinary tract disorders, emotional problems.
   2. THERAPY: Spiritual healing techniques: charismatic, polarity therapy; natural healing techniques, especially hydrotherapy.

D. *Health Maintenance*
   1. HERBS: Water plants: mosses, ferns, seaweeds (dulse, kelp, and so on) / borage
   2. VITAMINS: B complex, especially $B_2$, $B_3$ (niacin), and $B_{12}$ / vitamin C
   3. CELL SALTS: sodium sulfate (NAT-SULPH) / sodium phosphate (NAT-PHOS)
   4. MINERALS: iodine
   5. DIETARY NEEDS: almonds / beef / carrots / cucumbers / liver / lima beans / melon (all kinds) / squash

### no. 12 The Hanged Man

A. *Characteristics*
   1. TOTAL ESSENCE: transition, which in our time is from the Piscean to the Aquarian Age.
   2. ZODIAC SIGN: Pisces
   3. PLANET: Neptune
   4. COLOR: dark purple
   5. MUSICAL NOTE: low A
   6. FREQUENCY: 415.3 cps

B. *Themes for Personal Development*

  1. SOUL EXPRESSION: to transcend and sacrifice oneself and so reveal the laws that bring about transition.

  2. HUMAN EXPRESSION: the sacrifice of the animal aspect of one's nature in order to devote oneself to cosmic consciousness. This does not mean that a person with this card number should give up his or her animal nature; it means to give up the values that are exclusively associated with it and so integrate one's lower and higher natures.

C. *Common Disorders*

  1. GENERAL AILMENTS:

    a. Mucous discharge: asafetida / balm of Gilead / bloodroot / castor oil / flaxseed / gum arabic / licorice / manna / mullein root (boil with milk) / olive oil

    b. Poor circulation, cold extremities: balsam of Peru / black ash / black cohosh / cayenne pepper / hayflower / *indigo weed / kola nuts / sacred bark / shave grass / sweet marjoram / wahoo

    c. Weakness from poor bone structure in feet: carrageen / meadowsweet / nettles / sweet flag root / toadflax

  2. INFLUENCES ON PISCES:

    a. Squaring with Gemini:
    For chest weakness: borage / comfrey root and leaves / fireweed / garlic / hyssop / *poison hemlock / ribwort / sundew / sweet gum / wild cherry bark / *wild ipecac

    b. Opposing to Virgo:
    For intestinal disorders (digestive tract): aloes / blazing star / dwarf elder / goldenseal / peppermint / Peruvian bark / swamp milkweed / turtlehead / yarrow

    c. Squaring with Sagittarius:
    For liver trouble: culver's root / fringe-tree bark / liverwort / Oregon graperoot / *wild ipecac
    For gout: broom tops / club moss / garden sage / gravelroot / liferoot / meadow anemone / pareira root / Virginia snakeroot

D. *Health Maintenance*

  1. HERBS: all mosses, ferns, seaweeds (dulse, kelp, and so on). Ferns have negative ions and maintain tranquillity, as is true of green plants in general, especially pale green plants.

  2. VITAMINS: E, C, and D

  3. CELL SALTS: iron phosphate (FER-PHOS)

  4. MINERALS: iodine

5. DIETARY NEEDS: almonds / beef liver / cucumber / egg yolk / fish (especially mackerel, tuna, herring) / lettuce / lima beans / spinach / sweetbreads / wheatgrass / all seeds / all green leafy vegetables
6. ELEMENTS AND/OR TRACE ELEMENTS: bismuth: stimulant for parathyroids / lead: depressant for thyroid / polonium: hemostatic, astringent, respiratory depressant

## no. 13 Death

### A. Characteristics

1. TOTAL ESSENCE: the sign of regeneration, for every death is a prelude to rebirth.
2. ZODIAC SIGN: Aries
3. PLANET: Mars
4. COLOR: light red
5. MUSICAL NOTE: high C
6. FREQUENCY: 523.3 cps

### B. Themes for Personal Development

1. SOUL EXPRESSION: the perpetual movement in the universe through creation and destruction.
2. HUMAN EXPRESSION: ascension into the higher spheres of expression, heightening of the mental and spiritual faculties, increased sense perception, capacity to be hyperaesthetic.

### C. Common Disorders

1. GENERAL AILMENTS:
   a. Mucous discharge and head colds: boneset / coltsfoot / hollyhock / marshmallow root
   b. Nervousness: chamomile / licorice root / linden flowers / passionflower / *rhubarb root / slippery elm / valerian root / wood betony
   c. Tired eyes: eyebright / fennel / cucumber slices (apply to eyelids)
2. INFLUENCES ON ARIES:
   a. Squaring with Cancer:
      For stomach disorders: caraway seeds / ginseng / myrrh / yarrow
   b. Opposing to Libra:
      For kidney disorders: buchu leaves and root / gravelroot / juniper berries / parsley / shave grass / upland cranberry

c. Squaring with Capricorn:
   For skin disorders: chickweed / yellow dock

D. *Health Maintenance*

1. HERBS: aloes / barberry / broom tops / bryonia / catmint /
   cayenne pepper / coriander / crowfoot / cubebs / female fern /
   garlic / gentian / hawthorne / heal-all / *hemp / holy thistle /
   honeysuckle / hops / leeks / male fern / masterwort / nettles
   / onions / radishes / *rhubarb root / sweet basil / upland
   cranberry / valerian / *wormwood / yellow mustard

2. VITAMINS: A, B, and C

3. CELL SALTS: iron phosphate (FER-PHOS) and potassium
   phosphate (KALI-PHOS)

4. MINERALS: potassium

5. DIETARY NEEDS: bananas / beets / cabbage / carrots / celery /
   cheese / cod-liver oil / green beans / lemons / liver / milk
   (whole) / oranges / parsley / peas / red-colored fruits /
   spinach / sprouted greens / sweet potatoes / walnuts

6. ELEMENTS AND/OR TRACE ELEMENTS: calcium: for nerve
   insulation, nails, hair, teeth, and so on / lithium: diuretic,
   stimulant (found in dulse and kelp) / potassium: nervine /
   rubidium: diuretic, stimulant; removes uric acid (found in
   mineral springwater) / strontium: energizer (found mostly in
   red beets)

## no. 14 *Temperance*

A. *Characteristics*

1. TOTAL ESSENCE: regeneration; to take something out of form, fire
   it, and mold it to fulfill its role; so it is with the tempering of
   intellect to comprehend truth.

2. ZODIAC SIGN: Taurus

3. PLANET: Venus

4. COLOR: dark yellow

5. MUSICAL NOTE: low E

6. FREQUENCY: 311.1 cps

B. *Themes for Personal Development*

1. SOUL EXPRESSION: perpetual motion in our environment, com-
   bining the forces of nature and matter through the creation of
   concepts, bringing them into form; a passing state of energy.
   Thus, everything that is matter can be called spirit, but not everything that is spirit can be called matter.

2. HUMAN EXPRESSION: the regeneration of spirit (pure energy), with heightening of the tactile sense; intuition through touch. This transmutation of light into fire and fire into light is accomplished by the heart chakra.

C. *Common Disorders*

1. GENERAL AILMENTS:
   a. Throat afflictions: flaxseed / honey / horehound / licorice root / slippery elm bark / wild ginger
   b. Thyroid and goiter problems: Kelp (a seaweed) and Irish moss are for hyperthyroid conditions, acting as depressants; dulse (a seaweed) is for hypothyroid, acting as a stimulant.
   c. Thymus and lymph glands (affected if the person is not expressing him/herself): cayenne pepper / daisy / dandelion root / flaxseed / *Indian tobacco (mix with cayenne) / larkspur / lily root / myrtle / spinach leaves
   d. Obesity and edema: dogbane / pokeberries

2. INFLUENCES ON TAURUS:
   a. Squaring with Leo:
      For heart troubles (including dizziness and fainting): coriander seeds / culver's root / *foxglove / khella / lavender
   b. Opposing to Scorpio:
      For elimination troubles, bladder disorders: buckthorn / marshmallow root / parsley / *poison hemlock / yellow parilla
   c. Squaring with Aquarius:
      For blood impurities: coneflower / New Jersey tea / pokeroot
      For poor circulation: juniper berries / yellow parilla

D. *Health Maintenance*

1. HERBS: angelica / artichoke / birch / black alder / burdock / California poppy / catnip / club moss / coltsfoot / cowslip / cranesbill / daisy / dandelion root / devil's bit / figwort / flaxseed / *foxglove / kidneywort / lady's bedstraw / larkspur / lily root / marshmallow / mugwort / myrtle / *pennyroyal / plantain / privet / spinach leaves / thyme / wild cherry / yarrow
2. VITAMINS: A and E
3. CELL SALTS: sodium sulfate (NAT-SULPH)
4. MINERALS: Copper (found in the foods listed below and in apricot pits)

5. DIETARY NEEDS: apricots / beets / broccoli / endive / leafy vegetables / liver oils (as in cod liver) / mustard greens / parsley / seafoods / spinach / turnips / vegetable oils / watercress

6. ELEMENTS AND/OR TRACE ELEMENTS: aluminum: respiratory stimulant / antimony: parathyroid depressant / calcium: skeletal builder / copper: anticolic, antianemic / selenium: carminative / silicon: blood purifier, stomachic, hair builder / xenon: lung regenerative

## no. 15 The Devil

### A. Characteristics

1. TOTAL ESSENCE: to make things transparent in order to know the truth behind apparent multiplicity, and it is the Devil who stands in the light so we cannot see the truth.
2. ZODIAC SIGN: none
3. PLANET: Saturn
4. COLOR: indigo
5. MUSICAL NOTE: A
6. FREQUENCY: 440 cps

### B. Themes for Personal Development

1. SOUL EXPRESSION: predestination; the mystery of overcoming the self by understanding the higher self.
2. HUMAN EXPRESSION: to experience self through the means of one's physical vehicle and to manifest all the substances of the cosmos in a progressive manner.

### C. Common Disorders

1. GENERAL AILMENTS: glandular disorders of the endocrine system: gonads, adrenals, pancreas, thymus, thyroid, pituitary, pineal.
2. THERAPY: all naturopathic therapies: physiotherapy, hydrotherapy, herbology, biochemicals, and so on.

### D. Health Maintenance

1. HERBS: aconite / beet roots / *belladonna / common ivy / false hellebore / holly / *indigo weed / mullein / *poison hemlock / quince
2. VITAMINS: Vitamin B Complex
3. CELL SALTS: calcium phosphate (CALC-PHOS)
4. MINERALS: lead
5. DIETARY NEEDS: beef / black-eyed peas / cheeses / eggs /

fish / green-leaved vegetables / kidney / milk / nuts / seeds / soybeans / sweetbreads

6. ELEMENTS AND/OR TRACE ELEMENTS: cesium: antipruritic / indium: diaphoretic / oxygen: vermifuge, anodyne, demulcent, vitality builder

## no. 16 The Tower

A. *Characteristics*

1. TOTAL ESSENCE: the removal of all physical obstacles that inhibit growth.
2. ZODIAC SIGN: none
3. PLANET: Mars
4. COLOR: red
5. MUSICAL NOTE: middle C
6. FREQUENCY: 261.2 cps

B. *Themes for Personal Development*

1. SOUL EXPRESSION: the overcoming of physical obstacles, of pride, and of mental exhaustion, thereby penetrating the cosmic mysteries through the intuitive process.
2. HUMAN EXPRESSION: to overcome material wants in order to give vigor to healthy desires and thereby to diminish all obstacles.

C. *Common Disorders*

1. GENERAL AILMENTS: Nervous and intestinal disorders.
2. THERAPY: thermal therapeutics: diathermy machines and so on; creative meditation; mental imagery, such as guided reveries

D. *Health Maintenance*

1. HERBS: basil / bayberry / broom tops / garlic / wood betony
2. VITAMINS: $B_1$, $B_2$, $B_6$, and C
3. CELL SALTS: potassium phosphate (KALI-PHOS)
4. MINERALS: iron
5. DIETARY NEEDS: acerola cherries / almonds / apples / citrus fruits / endive / grapes / lettuce / red beets / spinach
6. ELEMENTS AND/OR TRACE ELEMENTS: calcium: for nerve insulation, nails, hair, teeth, and so on / lithium: diuretic, stimulant (found in dulse and kelp) / potassium: nervine / rubidium: diuretic, stimulant; removes uric acid (found in mineral springwater) / strontium: energizer (found mostly in red beets)

*no. 17 The Star*

A. *Characteristics*

  1. TOTAL ESSENCE: supernal powers, intuition, balancing the above and the below.

  2. ZODIAC SIGN: Gemini

  3. PLANET: Mercury

  4. COLOR: light violet

  5. MUSICAL NOTE: high B

  6. FREQUENCY: 493.9 cps

B. *Themes for Personal Development*

  1. SOUL EXPRESSION: the comprehension and perception of supernal powers and inner light, heightened perception, immortality.

  2. HUMAN EXPRESSION: heightening of the inner and outer vision to comprehend intuitively perceived images and to learn their practical applications.

C. *Common Disorders*

  1. GENERAL AILMENTS:

    a. Neuroses and nervous disorders, arising from failure to stabilize energies: bugleweed / ginseng / meadow saffron / scullcap / white cohosh
   *Indian tobacco (always use with cayenne pepper)

    b. Bronchial disorders: aconite / fireweed / skunk cabbage / spikenard

    c. Pulmonary disorders: lungwort / pleurisy root / ribwort / squill

    d. Anemia: black raspberry / passionflower / red raspberry / unicorn root

  2. INFLUENCES ON GEMINI:

    a. Squaring with Virgo:
   For intestinal and digestive disorders: black cohosh / bryonia / caraway seeds / garlic / goldenseal / wahoo

    b. Opposing to Sagittarius:
   For arthritis and rheumatism: black cohosh / *rhubarb root / sarsaparilla / sassafras / wintergreen
   For liver malfunction: Oregon graperoot / upland cranberry
   Or this formula, with doctor's supervision only: 1/4 tsp *mandrake root, 1/2 tsp *queen's-root, 1/2 tsp *wild ipecac, 1/2 tsp upland cranberry.

    c. Squaring with Pisces:

For colds and mucous discharge: coltsfoot / ginger / lemon /
mullein

D. *Health Maintenance*
   1. HERBS: celery / couch grass / endive / horehound / lavender /
      licorice / *mandrake / mulberry / parsnip / privet / savory /
      *tansy / valerian / vervain / wild carrot / *woodbine / yarrow
   2. VITAMINS: $B_3$ (niacin), $B_6$, $B_{12}$, C, D, and E
   3. CELL SALTS: potassium chloride (KALI-MUR)
   4. MINERALS: mercury
   5. DIETARY NEEDS: almonds / celery / corn / fish / lean meats /
      lemons / milk / oranges / parsley / spinach / strawberries /
      turnips
   6. ELEMENTS AND/OR TRACE ELEMENTS: actinium: spleen
      stimulant / cobalt: cardiac depressant / gallium: lymph
      depressant / radon: motor depressant; builds white blood
      cells   (All these are present in red beets.)

## no. 18 The Moon

A. *Characteristics*
   1. TOTAL ESSENCE: the reflection of wisdom upon the earth. (See
      "Total essence," card no. 2.)
   2. ZODIAC SIGN: Cancer
   3. PLANET: Moon
   4. COLOR: green
   5. MUSICAL NOTE: F
   6. FREQUENCY: 349.2 cps

B. *Themes for Personal Development*
   1. SOUL EXPRESSION: to remove the veils that shroud wisdom; the
      veils are woven from ignorance, lack of awareness, and lack of
      discipline.
   2. HUMAN EXPRESSION: spiritual integration and communication.
      Preserving one's life forces by integrating the higher and lower
      consciousness; perception and interpretation of widsom from
      higher sources.

C. *Common Disorders*
   1. GENERAL AILMENTS:
      a. Poor digestion: aniseseed / bay leaves / celery seeds /
         cinnamon bark / gingerroot / peppermint / Peruvian bark
      b. Dropsy (fluid edema, retention of water around the heart):
         dandelion / dwarf elder
      c. Hypersensitivity: balm / catnip / yellow lady's-slipper

2. INFLUENCES ON CANCER:
   a. Squaring with Libra:
      For kidney malfunction: corn silk / juniper berries
   b. Opposing to Capricorn:
      For skin disorders: chickweed / shepherd's purse / yellow dock
      For general debility: dandelion root / nettles / plantain root
   c. Squaring with Aries:
      For head colds: asafetida / coltsfoot / comfrey root (ground) / maidenhair fern
      For weak eyes: eyebright / fennel

D. *Health Maintenance*
   1. HERBS: water plants (such as watermelon) / cabbage / cucumbers / mouse-ear / pumpkin / rosemary / squash / water lily / willow
   2. VITAMINS: $B_2$, C, and E
   3. CELL SALTS: calcium fluoride (CALC-FLUOR)
   4. MINERALS: calcium
   5. DIETARY NEEDS: kale / lemons / milk / raisins / rye (in bread) / watercress / wild rice (with mushrooms and safflower oil)
   6. ELEMENTS AND/OR TRACE ELEMENTS: barium: stimulant for pituitary gland (use barium carbonate of the cell salts) / chlorine: disinfectant / nitrogen: purifier / radium: antiseptic / tellurium: internal detergent / thallium: germicide; muscle and tissue builder

## no. 19 The Sun

A. *Characteristics*
   1. TOTAL ESSENCE: regeneration of energies.
   2. ZODIAC SIGN: Leo
   3. PLANET: Sun
   4. COLOR: light orange
   5. MUSICAL NOTE: high D
   6. FREQUENCY: 314 cps

B. *Themes for Personal Development*
   1. SOUL EXPRESSION: expression of the higher energies, through joy and bliss. Achieved by organic alchemy, wherein the heart chakra unites inspiration (the white light from above) and the happiness of good physical condition.
   2. HUMAN EXPRESSION: through inspiration, to become the axis of

individual creative solar systems, to supply the energies needed by others, to radiate with complete indiscrimination toward all life.

C. *Common Disorders*
1. GENERAL AILMENTS:
   a. Heart problems (heart disease, fainting, and nervousness): coriander seeds / lavender / pimpernel / sweet basil / valerian
   b. Weak eyes: dill / plantain / watercress (as a compress made from a tea)
   c. Fevers: linden flowers / *pennyroyal
   d. Nausea and flatulence, gas: cinnamon / nutmeg / red sandalwood / rosemary
   e. Throat and bronchial disorders: chlorophyll / hawthorn / passionflower
      licorice root (use chamomile to cut its sweetness if necessary)
2. INFLUENCES ON LEO:
   a. Squaring with Scorpio:
      For better elimination: barberry / buckthorn / psyllium seeds
   b. Opposing to Aquarius:
      For blood disorders: burdock / restharrow / sassafras / yellow dock
   c. Squaring with Taurus:
      For laryngitis: liquid chlorophyll / flaxseed / quince seed / slippery elm
      For tonsillitis: liquid chlorophyll / licorice root / slippery elm

D. *Health Maintenance*
1. HERBS: almonds / bay leaves / celandine / centaury / chamomile / daisy / fennel / juniper / marigold / *mistletoe / olives / parsley seeds and leaves / *rhubarb root / saffron / Saint-John's-wort / sunflower
2. VITAMINS: C and E
3. CELL SALTS: magnesium phosphate (MAG-PHOS) (distributes electrical energy throughout the body)
4. MINERALS: gold (found especially in root vegetables such as beets, rutabagas, turnips, and shave grass root)
5. DIETARY NEEDS: barley / blueberry / citrus fruits (but bad for arthritis) / dulse (for underactive thyroids) / eggs / green

beans / kelp (for overactive thyroids) / lettuce / nuts / rice / seafood / seeds

6. ELEMENTS AND/OR TRACE ELEMENTS: cerium: cerebral stimulant / gold: thymus stimulant / iodine: antacid / iron: alterative, oxidizer / silver: laxative / sulfur: expectorant / titanium: bone builder / uranium and vanadium: stimulate pineal gland (found in root vegetables, volcanic ash, shellfish)

## no. 20 Judgment

### A. Characteristics

1. TOTAL ESSENCE: the awakener of souls from ignorance to consciousness.
2. ZODIAC SIGN: none
3. PLANET: Moon
4. COLOR: kelly green
5. MUSICAL NOTE: F
6. FREQUENCY: 349.2 cps

### B. Themes for Personal Development

1. SOUL EXPRESSION: awareness of immortality and judgment through consciousness.
2. HUMAN EXPRESSION: to elevate oneself to higher consciousness, attain self-consciousness; discovery of the now, rather than living in the past and fearing the future.

### C. Common Disorders

1. GENERAL AILMENTS:
   a. Female gynecological problems: cucumber / licorice root / madonna / white lily
   b. Fluid retention: Use diuretics (see Appendix A, part 1).
2. Therapy: Hydrotherapies (such as alternate hot and cold baths) / physiotherapies (massage) / polarity therapy.

### D. Health Maintenance

1. HERBS: cabbage / chickweed / cleavers / cucumbers / lettuce / lily / privet / sweet flag root / water lily / willow
2. VITAMINS: A, B, and C
3. CELL SALTS: All 12 Bioplasm salts
4. MINERALS: silver
5. DIETARY NEEDS: cabbage / cucumbers / green-leaved vegetables / melons / whole grains
6. ELEMENTS AND/OR TRACE ELEMENTS: barium: stimulant for pituitary gland (use Barium Carbonate of the cell salts) /

chlorine: disinfectant / nitrogen: purifier / radium: antiseptic
tellurium: internal detergent / thallium: germicide, muscle
and tissue builder

## no. 21 *The World*

A. *Characteristics*
1. TOTAL ESSENCE: bringer of renewal.
2. ZODIAC SIGN: none
3. PLANET: Sun
4. COLOR: Orange
5. MUSICAL NOTE: D
6. FREQUENCY: 293.7 cps

B. *Themes for Personal Development*
1. SOUL EXPRESSION: expression of the higher hierarchies, the triumph of adaptation of the self to these higher hierarchies.
2. HUMAN EXPRESSION: transformation and union of the soul essence with physical experience by mastery of the human ego.

C. *Common Disorders*
1. GENERAL AILMENTS:
   a. Heart weakness and incapacity to generate heat: birch bark / carrot tops / cayenne / centaury / chamomile / comfrey root / cough grass / oak bark
   b. Hypoglycemia: Check for copper content, iron assimilation for proper oxygen and glucose supply. / agar-agar / dandelion / devil's bit / dulse / kelp / liverwort / nettle / sorrel
2. THERAPY: Light and color therapies.

D. *Health Maintenance*
1. HERBS: almond / angelica / bay leaves / centaury / celandine / chamomile / colchicum root / eyebright / frankincense / garden rue / juniper berries / *mistletoe / mustards / pimpernel / Saint-John's-wort / sundew / sunflower seeds
2. VITAMINS: A and D
3. CELL SALTS: magnesium phosphate (MAG-PHOS)
4. MINERALS: gold
5. DIETARY NEEDS: Greenleaf vegetables / apricots / grains / wheat germ
6. ELEMENTS AND/OR TRACE ELEMENTS: cerium: cerebral stimulant / gold: thymus stimulant / iodine: antacid / iron: alterative, oxidizer / silver: laxative / sulfur: expectorant /

titanium: bone builder / uranium and Vanadium: stimulate pineal gland (found in root vegetables, volcanic ash, shellfish)

## no. 22 The Fool

### A. Characteristics

1. TOTAL ESSENCE: the all-encompassing light; symbol of the highest level of consciousness; harmony. The Fool knows what he is about; it is others who are fools for not recognizing him. A master card.
2. ZODIAC SIGN: none
3. PLANET: Pluto
4. COLOR: ultraviolet
5. MUSICAL NOTE: music of the spheres
6. FREQUENCY: none

### B. Themes for Personal Development

1. SOUL EXPRESSION: recognition of the inner source, the divine self.
2. HUMAN EXPRESSION: freedom from external authority; action based on inner authority, inner knowing.

### C. Common Disorders

1. GENERAL AILMENTS: ailments of any kind arising from individual's failing to express inner knowing. Choose remedies as described elsewhere in this book for specific ailments.
2. THERAPY: stellar healing, astrological medicine, the attracting of forces from the different planets. The body must be in top shape to fulfill the mission of this card.

### D. Health Maintenance

Voluntary control to the utmost; listening to the body and interpreting of its needs. The reason there are no specific recommendations for health maintenance is that once we reach optimal voluntary control (holistic health); our bodies will direct us to our needs and no added herbs, vitamins, cell salts, or special dietary needs will be necessary. For example, the author himself uses none of the ingredients described in this book because of his recognized voluntary control.

# Appendix A:
# A Guide to Medicinal Herbs

## Introduction

This appendix is designed to be used in conjunction with the general discussion of the use of herbs in Chapter 5 and with the discussion of the tarot system of healing (Chapter 6), in which herbal remedies are indicated for specific conditions or for certain types of people.

Before using any of the herbs, be sure to read the directions for the preparation of herbal teas in Chapter 5.

An asterisk (*) indicates that an herb is *toxic*. Use an alternative herb if there is one. Otherwise, use no more than a knife's point of the substance, and never use it alone; it must always be mixed with other appropriate herbs, as described in Chapter 5. Do not use a toxic herb regularly except under a doctor's prescription.

Unless otherwise stated (e.g., if bark, root, or stem is specified), an herb means the leaves (and flowers).

Part 1 of this appendix arranges the herbs according to therapeutic applications, which are listed alphabetically. Many of these therapeutic terms may be unfamiliar to you; after each term, you will find its definition. Part 2 lists the herbs alphabetically, giving the therapeutic applications for each. If you do not understand the meaning of a therapeutic term, look it up in Part 1.

## Part 1: Therapeutic Applications

ABORTIFACIENTS: *abortion-producing agents* / cotton-root bark

ABSORBENTS: *agents capable of absorption* / charcoal

ALKALIZERS: *alkaline-rendering agents* / lemon

**ALTERATIVES:** *altering and improving the nutritive processes and other functions of the body* / American elder / American saffron / barberry / black alder / black cohosh / *blue flag root / burdock / butternut / carob tree / chlorophyll / cod-liver oil / common alder / coneflower / dandelion / dogwood / dwarf elder / *eagle vine bark / elecampane root / goldenseal / *indigo weed / kelp / leafcup, bears-foot (American) / manaca / meadow anemone / mountain laurel / New Jersey tea / Oregon grape / pipsissewa / pokeroot / prickly ash / queen's-root / red clover / rheum (rhubarb) root / Saint-John's-wort / sassafras / spikenard / stoneroot / tiger lily / turkey corn / vervain / violet / yellow dock / yellow parilla

**AMYLOLYTICS:** *converting starch into sugar* / diastase

**ANALGESICS:** *pain relievers* / Jamaica dogwood / meadow saffron / Peruvian bark / wintergreen

**ANAPHRODISIACS:** *sex depressants* / hops

**ANESTHETICS:** *causing insensibility* / menthol

**ANHYDROTICS:** (ANTISUDORIFICS) *perspiration-checking agents* / burr (also called broad-burused, spring clot bur) / daisy / white agaric

**ANODYNES:** *pain relievers* / aconite / black cohosh / bryonia / cayenne / cloves / corn silk / creosote (obtained from wood tar) / *hemp / *henbane leaves / hops / *jimsonweed / lettuce opium / meadow anemone / motherwort / pareira root / peppermint / quaking aspen / rheum (rhubarb) root / yellow clover

**ANTHELMINTICS:** *expelling intestinal worms* / Carolina pink / female fern / garden rue / horsemint / male fern / pleurisy root / pomegranate root bark / satonica / *tansy / thyme oil / turpentine, oil of / white cohosh / *wormwood

**ANTIARTERIOSCLEROTICS:** *preventing hardening of the arteries* / garden rue

**ANTIBIOTICS:** *antibacterial agents* / bromelin / coneflower / Peruvian bark

**ANTICATARRHALS:** *preventing inflammation of mucous membranes* / asafetida / balm of Gilead / bloodwort / castor oil / coltsfoot / comfrey root / ginger / gum arabic / hollyhock / lemon / marshmallow root / mullein / olive oil / saw palmetto

**ANTIHEMORRHAGICS:** *arresting bleeding* / buckthorn / shepherd's purse / witch hazel

**ANTIMALARIALS:** *alleviating or curing malaria* / Peruvian bark (quinine)

**ANTINAUSEANTS:** *alleviating or curing nausea* / cinnamon / nutmeg / red sandalwood / rosemary

**ANTIPERIODICS:** *preventive of regular recurrences of a disease such as malaria* / black willow / dogwood / eucalyptus (blue gum) / Peruvian bark (quinine) / sweet flag / wahoo / white agaric

**ANTIPHLOGISTICS:** *preventing inflammations* / flaxseed / garlic / *Indian tobacco / onion / sulfonated hydrocarbons

ANTIPRURITICS: *preventing or relieving itching* / camphor

ANTIPYRETICS: *fever-reducing agents* / aconite / pareira root / wintergreen

ANTIRHEUMATICS: *relieving or preventing rheumatism* / black cohosh / bryonia / California buckthorn / chamomile / dulse / lavender / lungwort / meadow saffron / Peruvian bark / rheum (rhubarb) root / sarsaparilla / sassafras / wintergreen

ANTISCORBUTICS: *counteracting scurvy* / lemon / shepherd's purse / watercress

ANTISEPTICS: *agents having destructive action on microorganisms of disease, decay, or fermentation* / aconite / buchu / camphor / cankerroot / coneflower / copaiba / creosote / elecampane root / eucalyptus / guaiac wood / hemlock / juniper-tar oil / kavakava / large flowering spurge / menthol / myrrh / pale catechu / pine tar / ribwort / santal oil / smooth sumac / sweet gum / thuja / thyme oil / turpentine, oil of / upland cranberry / Vaseline / wintergreen

ANTISPASMODICS: *relieving spasms, checking convulsions* / asafetida / black cohosh / black haw / blackthorn root / blue cohosh / camphor / Carolina jasmine / cayenne pepper / colicroot / cuminseed and fruit / daisy / garden rue / ginger / gravelweed / green hellebore / *henbane / horse nettle / *Indian tobacco (always use with cayenne pepper as demulcent) / *jimsonweed / khella / larkspur / motherwort / muskroot / passionflower / *pennyroyal / pill-bearing spurge / *poison hemlock / prickly ash / red clover / shave grass / skullcap / skunk cabbage / spinach leaves / sunflower seeds / valerian / vervain / *woodbine / yellow clover

ANTISYPHILITICS: *alleviating or curing syphilis* / dandelion / manaca

ANTITHROMBICS: *checking coagulation, counteracting blood clotting* / yellow clover

ANTITUSSIVES: *cough-relieving agents* / black cohosh / burdock / chestnut / coltsfoot / horsemint / lungwort / mullein / red clover

APERIENTS: *mild cathartics (purgatives)* / aloes / couch grass / dandelion

AROMATICS: *imparting a fragrant smell* / chamomile / daisy / huckleberry / marigold / marjoram / passionflower / sassafras / white rose / wild thyme

ASTRINGENTS: *agents producing contraction of tissues* / agrimony / American elder / balm / bayberry / black alder / black raspberry / blackthorn berries / black willow / bramble / bugleweed / button snakeroot / Canada fleabane / cankerroot / chestnut / cinnamon / common alder / cranesbill / cubebs / elecampane root / eyebright / fragrant sumac / goldenseal / hemlock / horse chestnut / kino / large flowering spurge lily root / liverwort / mango / marshmallow / matico leaves / mountain laurel / myrrh / nettles / New Jersey tea / nutgalls / oil of Copaiba / pale catechu / peach tree leaves / pichi / privet / red raspberry / rhatany / *rhubarb root / ribwort / Saint-John's-wort / santal oil / shave grass / shepherd's purse / shinleaf / smooth sumac / Solomon's seal / squaw vine /

stavesacre / stoneroot / touch-me-not / upland cranberry / Virginia stonecrop / wafer ash / white hellebore / white oak bark / wickup / wild cherry bark / witch hazel / yarrow / yerba mansa / yerba reuma

BASES: *principal ingredient of a compound* / resin

BITTERS: *bitter-tasting tonic or stomachic* / American columbo

BRONCHODILATORS: *enlarger of bronchial tubes* / *belladonna

CARDIAC DEPRESSANTS: *depressants of hyperactive heart* / *fly agaric / male fern

CARDIAC STIMULANTS: *stimulating underactive heart* / cactus / Canadian hemp / quebracho / strophanthus (tincture) / *wormwood

CARDIANTS: *tonics for the heart* / broom tops / cayenne pepper / common milkweed / coriander seeds / *foxglove / khella / lavender / lily of the valley / squill / veronica / *wild geranium root

CARMINATIVES: *relievers of flatulence or colic* / allspice / American elder / aniseseed / asafetida / bitter orange peel / black pepper / buchu / cajuput oil / caraway seed / cardamon seed / catnip / chamomile, German / chamomile, Roman / cinnamon / cloves / coriander seed / cubebs / cumin seeds and fruit / fennel / feverfew / fireweed / garden rue / garden sage / ginger / horsemint / lavender flowers / lemon / menthol / muskroot / nutmeg / parsley seeds / peach tree leaves / *pennyroyal / peppermint / prickly ash / red sandalwood / *rhubarb root / rosemary / sarsaparilla / sassafras / spearmint / sweet flag / sweet orange peel / white rose / wild ginger / wood betony / yerba mansa

CATHARTICS: *purging agents, purgatives* / bayberry / black ash / *blue flag / broom tops / bryonia / buckthorn / California buckthorn / Canadian hemp / couch grass / culver's root / horehound / kousso / large flowering spurge / mulberry / *queen's-root / *rhubarb root / sacred bark / senna / spoonwood / squirting cucumber / *wild ipecac

CHOLAGOGUES: *promoting the flow of bile* / culver's root / fringe tree / *mandrake root / *queen's-root / tetterwort / turtlehead

CHOLERETICS: *stimulating the secretion of bile by the liver* / *blue flag / cleavers / culver's root / dandelion root / liverwort / Oregon graperoot / *wild ipecac

CHOLERICS: *activating sluggish liver associated with slight jaundice or dyspepsia* / *wild ipecac

CONDIMENTS: *seasonings or relishes* / allspice / black pepper / garden sage / ginger / nutmeg / peppermint / spearmint / white mustard

CORONARY DILATORS: *enlarging the blood vessels of the heart* / coffee

CORRIGENTS: *tending to improve, modify, or counteract other unpleasant remedies* / cinnamon / fennel / lemon / *pennyroyal

COUNTERIRRITANTS: *producing surface inflammations in order to relieve deep-seated inflammations* / arnica / camphor / cayenne pepper / horsemint / turpentine, oil of / white mustard / wintergreen

CYCLOPLEGICS: *producing paralysis of the ciliary muscle of the eye* / *henbane

DEMULCENTS: *soothing, relieving irritations, especially of the mucous membranes and surfaces* / barley / coltsfoot / comfrey / couch grass / elm bark / flaxseed / gum arabic / honey / huckleberry / licorice root / lily root / manna / marshmallow / mullein / olive oil / sassafras / shepherd's purse / slippery elm / spermaceti

DEODORANTS: *neutralizers of offensive odors* / charcoal / chlorophyll / creosote / eucalyptus / thyme oil

DEPRESSANTS: *agents lowering nervous or functional activities* / aconite / arnica / *belladonna / calabar bean / camphor / Carolina jasmine / *fly agaric / garlic / green hellebore / *Indian tobacco / nutmeg / pheasant's-eye / poison ivy / *wormwood

DERMETICS: *for skin problems* / chickweed / comfrey / marjoram / shepherd's purse / yellow dock / Use Saint-John's-wort, sweet fern, heal-all and witch hazel together in a Vaseline base.

DETERGENTS: *cleansing or purging agents* / barberry / Oregon grape

DIAPHORETICS: *perspiration-causing agents* / aconite / American elder / American saffron / blue cohosh / boneset / bramble / burdock / cajuput oil / catnip / chamomile, German / chamomile, Roman / coralroot / dwarf elder / elecampane / *fly agaric / ginger / guaiac root / *hemp / holy thistle / horehound / horsemint / jaborandi / lemon / *pennyroyal / pleurisy root / prickly ash / sassafras / spikenard / vervain / Virginia snakeroot / wild ginger

DIGESTANTS: *promoting digestion* / aniseed / barberry / bay leaves / celery seeds / cinnamon bark / dwarf elder / garlic / gentian root / ginseng / hops / licorice root / myrrh / Oregon grape / papaya enzymes / peppermint / pepsin / slippery elm / swamp milkweed / wahoo / *wormwood

DISCUTIENTS: *agents dispersing or absorbing morbid tissue* / flaxseed / *Indian tobacco / *indigo weed / leafcup / yellow clover

DISINFECTANTS: *agents destroying germs causing disease* / thyme oil

DIURETICS: *agents promoting excretion of urine* / American elder / bayberry / *blue flag or iris / broom tops / buchu / burr / burdock / button snakeroot / cactus / Canadian hemp / caraway seeds / Christmas rose / cleavers / club moss / coffee / common milkweed / corn silk / couch grass / cucumber / daisy / dandelion / dwarf elder / *eagle vine bark / elecampane / fireweed / garden sage / gravelroot / gravelweed / guaiac wood / hollyhock / horehound / juniper berries / kavakava / lemon / liferoot / lily of the valley / manaca / meadow anemone / mullein leaves / nettle / pareira root / parsley seeds or leaves / pipsissewa / pumpkin seed /

quaking aspen / Saint-John's-wort / santonica / sassafras / saw palmetto / sevenbark / shave grass / shepherd's purse / sourwood / spearmint / squaw vine / squill / stoneroot / strophanthus seeds / swamp milkweed / thuja / unicorn root / upland cranberry / Virginia snakeroot / yarrow
All diuretics must contain at least these three ingredients: upland cranberry, juniper berries, and buchu leaves.

**DUSTING POWDERS:** *drying agents for local application* / club moss / marigold (borated) / spermaceti

**ECBOLICS:** *accelerating childbirth, abortion-producing agents* / cotton-root bark

**EMETICS:** *vomiting-causing agents* / *blue flag / boneset / butternut / horehound / *Indian tobacco / *indigo weed / ipecac / large flowering spurge / squill / white mustard

**EMETOCATHARTICS:** *agents with emetic and purgative qualities* / *indigo weed / pokeroot / spoonwood / yellow parilla

**EMMENAGOGUES:** *agents promoting menstrual flow* / aloes / American saffron / balm / black cohosh / blue cohosh / button snakeroot / Christmas rose / corn smut / cotton-root bark / ergot / feverfew / liferoot / meadow anemone / motherwort / parsley seeds / *pennyroyal / saffron / spinach leaves / *tansy / thuja / turpentine, oil of / white cohosh / wild ginger / wild thyme / wood betony / yarrow

**EMOLLIENTS:** *softening and soothing agents, especially for mucous membranes* / cacao butter / castor oil / elm bark / flaxseed / hollyhock / lard / olive oil / slippery elm / spermaceti / Vaseline / wool fat

**EMULSIFIERS:** *agents effecting emulsification of oils* / burdock root / elder root / gum arabic / hollyhock

**EXCITANTS:** *stimulating agents* / sweet flag

**EXPECTORANTS:** *expellants of saliva, mucus, and other materials from lungs and windpipe* / asafetida / balsam of Peru / black cohosh / bloodroot / cajuput oil / Carolina pink / coltsfoot / creosote / cubebs / elecampane / fireweed / garlic / guaiac wood / gum plant / hemlock / horehound / *Indian tobacco / ipecac / kavakava / lemon / licorice root / liverwort / lungwort / manna / mullein / nettles / onion / pill-bearing spurge / pine tar / senega / skunk cabbage / spikenard / squill / sundew / sweet gum / turpentine, oil of / violet / Virginia snakeroot / wild cherry bark / wild ginger / *wild ipecac / yerba santa

**FEBRIFUGES:** *fever-reducing agents* / black pepper / black willow / bryonia / green hellebore / lemon / linden flowers / mulberry / *pennyroyal / quaking aspen / vervain / *wormwood

**FLAVORING AGENTS:** *giving aroma and flavor to a remedy* / bitter orange peel / cardamon seed / fennel / lavender flowers / lemon / spearmint / sweet orange peel / wintergreen

**GERMICIDES:** *microbe-destroying agents* / kino

HEMOSTATICS: *agents arresting hemorrhages* / bugleweed / cinnamon / cranesbill / ergot / honey / mango / nutgalls / rhatany / turpentine, oil of / yarrow / yerba santa

HYDRAGOGUES: *producing discharge of watery fluid* / bitter apple / jalapa resin / *mandrake root / tetterwort

HYPNOTICS: *sleep-inducing agents* / bitter apple / *henbane / passionflower / *poison hemlock

INSECT REPELLANTS: *agents repelling insects* / *pennyroyal

IRRITANTS: *irritation-causing agents* / balsam of Peru / cloves / pine tar / sacred bark / squirting cucumber / thuja

LAXATIVES: *mild cathartics (purgatives of the bowels)* / American columbo / American saffron / boneset / buckthorn / butternut / flaxseed / honey / huckleberry / *indigo weed / licorice root / manna / olive oil / pansy stems and leaves / psyllium seeds / *rhubarb root / sacred bark / senna / Vaseline / yellow dock / yellow parilla

LENITIVES: *relieving discomfort due to dryness; demulcents* / barley / flaxseed / licorice root / marshmallow / slippery elm

LUBRICANTS: *lubricating agents* / agar-agar / lard / wool fat

MIOTICS: *agents causing contraction of the pupil and diminishing intra-ocular tension* / Calabar bean / *fly agaric / jaborandi

MOTOR EXCITANTS: *exciting the nerves or nerve centers transmitting impulses to any muscle* / Quaker buttons

MOTOR INHIBITORS: *restraining the chemical or physiological action of the nerves or nerve centers controlling muscles* / *belladonna

MOUTHWASHES: *for cleansing the mouth* / barberry

MUCILAGES: *vehicles acting as soothing agents to mucous surfaces* / gum arabic

MYDRIATICS: *agents causing dilation of the pupil* / *belladonna / *henbane / *jimsonweed

NARCOTICS: *agents causing drowsiness, stupor, or unconsciousness* / *belladonna / *blue flag root / Christmas rose / *hemp leaves / *henbane / Jamaica dogwood / *jimsonweed / *tansy / *wormwood

NERVINES: *nerve-calming agents* / asafetida / black cohosh / black haw / bloodroot / catnip / chamomile, German / chamomile, Roman / coriander seeds / *hemp / hops / lavender / linden flowers / meadow anemone / muskroot / oats / passionflower / red sandalwood / Saint-John's-wort / skullcap / spearmint / spinach leaves / valerian root / white cohosh / wood betony / yellow clover / yellow lady's-slipper

NUTRIENTS: *nutritive agents* / barley / cod-liver oil / honey / lemon / manna / oats / olive oil

OXYTOCICS: *labor-hastening agents* / Canadian fleabane / corn smut / ergot / *mistletoe / Peruvian bark

PARASITICIDES: *expelling parasites (intestinal)* / balsam of Peru / cajuput oil / chrysarobin powder / juniper-tar oil / nutmeg / pine tar / stavesacre

PARTURIENT PREPARATORS: *labor-preparing agents* / squaw vine

PERFUMES: *fragrances* / lavender flowers

PRESERVATIVES: *aiding the preservation of substances* / wintergreen

PROTECTIVES: *agents warding off infection* / cacao butter / club moss / Vaseline

PROTEOLYTIC ENZYMES: *promoting hydrolysis of proteins, splitting them into peptides and amino acids* / aloes / butternut / castor oil / Christmas rose / cotton oil / jalapa resin / *mandrake root / pokeroot

PURGATIVES: *cleansing, purifying agents* / broom tops / couch grass / female fern / pepsin / *rhubarb root / strawberry leaves and stems

PUSTULANTS: *causing production of pustules* / arnica / cotton oil

REFRIGERANTS: *agents causing cooling effect* / lemon / menthol

RELAXANTS: see *Sedatives*

RESPIRATORY STIMULANTS: *agents stimulating breathing* / quebracho

RESPIRATORY VASOCONSTRICTORS: *agents causing constriction of blood vessels of respiratory system* / jack-in-the-pulpit

REVULSANTS: *causing dilation of blood vessels* / cayenne pepper / garlic

RUBEFACIENTS: *causing mild irritation or reddening of skin* / camphor / cayenne pepper / garlic / ginger / horsemint / meadow saffron / menthol / onion / sassafras / tetterwort / white mustard / wintergreen

SECRETORY DEPRESSANTS: *depressing secretions* / *belladonna

SEDATIVES: *(relaxants) calming agents* / black cohosh / blackthorn root / bugleweed / chamomile / Carolina jasmine / corn silk / *henbane / hops / *jimsonweed / khella / lavender / lettuce opium / meadow anemone / mountain laurel / mullein / New Jersey tea / parsley / passionflower / pill-bearing spurge / *poison hemlock / red clover / Saint-John's-wort / saw palmetto / sevenbark / stavesacre / sundew / white hellebore / wild cherry bark / *woodbine / yarrow

SIALAGOGUES: *promoting saliva* / *fly agaric / jaborandi / prickly ash

STIMULANTS: *stimulating, augmenting function of any tissue* / aconite / agrimony / allspice / American columbo / arnica / balsam of Peru / bitter orange peel / black ash / black pepper / bloodroot / bryonia / buchu / butternut / button snakeroot / cactus / cajuput oil / Calabar bean / camphor / caraway seeds / Carolina jasmine / cayenne pepper / chamomile, German / Christmas rose / coffee / coriander seed / corn smut / dwarf elder / elder root / evening primrose / fennel / feverfew / garden rue / garden sage / garlic / ginger / ginseng / guarana / gum plant / hemlock / holy thistle / horehound / horsemint / *Indian tobacco / *indigo weed / juniper berries / kelp / kola nut / lavender flowers / leafcup / lemon / liferoot / marigold / matico leaves / menthol / *mistletoe / muskroot / myrrh / oats / Ohio buckeye / onion / parsley seed / *pennyroyal / peppermint / pleurisy root / poison ivy / radish / sacred bark / Saint-Ignatius's-bean / sassafras / senega root / shepherd's purse / spearmint / spikenard / sweet gum / sweet orange peel / *tansy / thuja / turpentine, oil of / Virginia snakeroot / water hemlock / white rose / wood betony / *wormwood / yellow lady's-slipper

STOMACHICS: *agents improving digestion and appetite* / aloes / American columbo / asafetida / bitterwood / blazing star / boneset / cajuput oil / caraway seed / cardamom seed / chamomile, Roman / cloves / coriander seed / cubebs / daisy / dandelion / dwarf elder / *eagle vine bark / elecampane / garlic / gentian root / ginseng / horehound / juniper berries / lemon / myrrh / Peruvian bark / Quaker buttons / swamp milkweed / turtlehead / wahoo / *wormwood / yarrow / yellow parilla / yerba santa

STYPTICS: *astringent, hemostatic (blood-stopping) agents* / buckthorn / witch hazel

SUDORIFICS: see *Diaphoretics*

TAENIACIDES: *agents that kill tapeworms* / kousso / turpentine, oil of

TAENIAFUGES: *expelling tapeworms* / spoonwood

TINEACIDES: *curing ringworm* / fishberries

TONICS: *raising mental or physical tone* / agrimony / American columbo / barberry / bayberry / bitter orange peel / bitterwood / black alder / black cohosh / black haw / black pepper / black raspberry / blazing star / blue cohosh / boneset / bramble / buchu / buckthorn / bugleweed / burr / button snakeroot / cankerroot / common alder / coneflower / coralroot / daisy / dandelion / dwarf elder / elecampane / feverfew / garden sage / gentian root / goldenseal / gravelroot / gravelweed / holy thistle / hops / horehound / kavakava / liferoot / marjoram / matico leaves / onion / Oregon grape / pansy / Peruvian bark / pipsissewa / prickly ash / Quaker buttons / quaking aspen / quinine / red raspberry / Saint-Ignatius's-bean / sarsaparilla / sassafras / saw palmetto / skullcap / Solomon's seal / stoneroot / sweet flag / sweet orange peel / tiger lily / turkey corn / unicorn root / upland cranberry / wafer ash / wahoo / wild cherry bark / *wormwood / wood betony / yellow dock / yellow parilla / yerba mansa / yerba santa

VAGINAL INHIBITORS: *restraining physiological or chemical action of vagina* / *belladonna

VASCULAR SEDATIVE: *calming of circulation* / bugleweed

VASOCONSTRICTORS: *constricting blood vessels* / eyebright / horse chestnut / pheasant's-eye

VASODILATORS: *enlarging blood vessels* / balsam of Peru / *belladonna /
bittersweet / black ash / *fly agaric / garlic / *indigo weed / juniper
berries / khella / kola nuts / sacred bark / shave grass / sweet marjoram /
white agaric / yellow parilla

VEHICLES: *carriers for dissolving of therapeutically active agents* / bee wax /
cacao butter / cardamom seed / eucalyptus / flaxseed / gentian root / gum
arabic / honey / lard / lemon / Vaseline / wool fat

VERMIFUGES:*expelling intestinal worms* / bitterwood / common milkweed /
feverfew / kousso / mulberry / pomegranate root bark / pumpkin seed /
spoonwood / thyme oil / turpentine, oil of / wormseed / *wormwood

VESICANTS: *agents that cause blistering when applied locally* / arnica /
croton oil / eucalyptus / tetterwort / white mustard

VULNERARIES: *agents that encourage and hasten healing of wounds* /
comfrey / marigold / myrrh / Saint-John's-wort / sulfonated hydrocarbons /
touch-me-not


## Part 2: List of Herbs and Their Uses

ACACIA: see *gum arabic*

ACONITE *(Aconitum):* anodyne / antipyretic / antiseptic / depressant /
diaphoretic / stimulant

AGAR-AGAR *(Agar):* lubricant

AGRIMONY *(Agrimonia):* astringent / stimulant / tonic

ALLSPICE *(Pimenta):* carminative / condiment / stimulant

ALOE *(Aloe):* aperient / emmenagogue / proteolytic / enzyme /
stomachic

AMERICAN COLUMBO *(Frasera):* bitters / laxative / stomachic

AMERICAN ELDER *(Sambucus):* alterative / astringent / carminative /
diaphoretic / diuretic

AMERICAN SAFFRON *(Carthamus):* alterative / diaphoretic / emmenagogue /
laxative

AMERICAN SENNA: see *senna*

ANISESEED *(Pimpinella anisum):* carminative / digestant

ARNICA *(Arnica;* also called *leopard's-bane):* counterirritant / depressant /
pustulant / stimulant / vesicant

ASAFETIDA *(Ferula assafoetida):* anticatarrhal / antispasmodic / carminative /
expectorant / nervine / stomachic

*ATROPINE: see *belladonna*

BALM *(Melissa officinalis):* astringent / emmenagogue / stimulant /
tonic

BALM OF GILEAD *(Populus candicans):* anticatarrhal

BALSAM OF PERU *(Balsamum peruvianum):* expectorant / irritant / parasiticide / stimulant / vasodilator

BARBERRY *(Berberis vulgaris):* alterative / detergent / digestant / mouthwash / tonic

BARLEY *(Hordeum):* demulcent / lenitive / nutrient

BAYBERRY *(Myrica):* astringent / cathartic / diuretic / tonic

BAY LEAVES *(Laurus):* digestant

*BELLADONNA *(Atropa;* also called *deadly nightshade;* source of atropine): bronchodilator (atropine) / depressant / motor inhibitor (atropine) / mydriatic (atropine) / narcotic / secretory depressant / vaginal inhibitor (atropine) / vasodilator (atropine)
(Toxic; never take without a doctor's prescription)

BITTER APPLE *(Citrullus colocynthis):* hydragogue / hypnotic

BITTER ORANGE PEEL *(Aurantii amari cortex):* carminative / flavoring agent / stimulant / tonic

BITTERSWEET *(Solanum dulcamara):* vasodilator

BITTERWOOD *(Quassia;* also called *quassia):* stomachic / tonic / vermifuge

BLACK ALDER *(Prinos verticillatos):* alterative / astringent / tonic

BLACK ASH *(Fraxinus):* cathartic / stimulant / vasodilator

BLACK COHOSH *(Cimicifuga;* also called *squawroot):* alterative / anodyne / antirheumatic / antispasmodic / antitussive / emmenagogue / expectorant / nervine / sedative / tonic

BLACK HAW *(Viburnum):* antispasmodic / nervine / tonic

BLACK PEPPER *(Piper nigrum):* carminative / condiment / febrifuge / stimulant / tonic

BLACK RASPBERRY *(Rubus villosus):* astringent / tonic

BLACKTHORN ROOT *(Prunus spinosa;* also called *sloe, wild plum):* antispasmodic / astringent (berries) / sedative

BLACK WILLOW *(Salix nigra):* antiperiodic / astringent / febrifuge

BLAZING STAR *(Aletris):* stomachic / tonic

BLOODROOT *(Sanguinaria):* expectorant / nervine / stimulant
(Also available in pellets as sanguinaria.)

BLOODWORT *(Polygonum hydropiper):* anticatarrhal

BLUE COHOSH *(Caulophyllum):* antispasmodic / diaphoretic / emmenagogue / tonic

*BLUE FLAG ROOT *(Iris;* also called iris): alterative / cathartic / choleretic / diuretic / emetic / narcotic

BLUE GUM: see *eucalyptus*

BONESET *(Eupatorium perfoliatum):* diaphoretic / emetic / laxative / stomachic / tonic

BRAMBLE *(Rubus fructicasus):* astringent / diaphoretic / tonic

BROMELIN (enzyme from pineapple): antibiotic

BROOM TOPS *(Cystisus scoparius):* cardiant / cathartic / diuretic / purgative (mix with dandelion)

BRYONIA *(Bryonia):* anodyne / antirheumatic / cathartic / febrifuge / stimulant

BUCHU *(Barosma):* antiseptic / carminative / diuretic / stimulant / tonic

BUCKTHORN *(Barosma betulina):* antihemorrhagic / cathartic / laxative / styptic / tonic

BUGLEWEED *(Lycopus):* astringent / hemostatic / sedative / tonic / vascular sedative

BURDOCK *(Arctium lappa):* alterative / antitussive / diaphoretic / diuretic / emulsifier (root)

BURR *(Xanthium spinosum):* anhydrotic / diuretic / tonic (Renal)

BUTTON SNAKEROOT *(Eryngium):* astringent / diuretic / emmenagogue / stimulant / tonic

CACAO BUTTER *(Oleum theobromatis):* emollient / protective / vehicle

CACTUS *(Cactus):* cardiac stimulant / diuretic / stimulant

CADE, OIL OF: see *Juniper*

CAJUPUT, OIL OF *(Melaleuca leucadendra):* carminative / diaphoretic / expectorant / parasiticide / stimulant / stomachic

CALABAR BEAN *(Physostigma):* depressant / miotic / stimulant

CALIFORNIA BUCKTHORN *(Rhamnus californica):* antirheumatic / cathartic

CAMPHOR: antipruritic / antiseptic / antispasmodic / counterirritant / depressant / rubefacient / stimulant

CANADA FLEABANE *(Erigeron):* astringent / oxytocic

CANADIAN HEMP *(Apocynum):* cardiac stimulant / cathartic / diuretic

CANKERROOT *(Coptis):* antiseptic / astringent / tonic

CARAWAY SEEDS *(Carum):* carminative / diuretic / stimulant / stomachic

CARDAMOM SEEDS *(Elettaria cardamomum):* carminative / flavoring agent / stomachic / vehicle

CAROBA *(Jacaranda frocera):* alterative

CAROLINA JASMINE *(Gelsemium):* antispasmodic / depressant / sedative / stimulant

CAROLINA PINK *(Spigelia):* anthelmintic / expectorant

CASTOR OIL *(Oleum ricini):* anticatarrhal (with olive oil) / emollient / proteolytic enzyme
(To lessen the strong taste, take a swallow of milk, and let it go down slowly to coat the throat.)

CATNIP *(Nepeta cataria):* carminative / diaphoretic / nervine

CAYENNE PEPPER *(Capsicum frutescens):* anodyne / antispasmodic / cardiant / counterirritant / revulsant / rubefacient / stimulant

CELERY SEEDS *(Apium):* digestant

CHAMOMILE, GERMAN *(Matricaria):* antirheumatic / aromatic / carminative / diaphoretic / nervine / sedative / stimulant

CHAMOMILE, ROMAN *(Anthemis):* antirheumatic / aromatic / carminative / diaphoretic / nervine / sedative / stomachic

CHARCOAL *(Carbo):* absorbent / deodorant

CHESTNUT *(Castanea):* antitussive / astringent

CHICKWEED *(Stellaria):* dermetic

CHLOROPHYLL: alterative / deodorant
(Can be obtained from comfrey, alfalfa, wheatgrass.)

CHRISTMAS ROSE *(Helleborus niger;* also called *black hellebore):* diuretic / emmenagogue / narcotic / proteolytic / enzyme / stimulant

CHRYSAROBIN POWDER *(Helleborus niger):* parasiticide

CINNAMON *(Cinnamomum):* antinauseant / astringent / carminative / corrigent / digestant / hemostatic

CLEAVERS *(Galium):* choleretic / diuretic

CLOVES *(Eugenia caryophyllata):* anodyne / carminative / irritant / stomachic

CLUB MOSS *(Lycopodium):* diuretic / dusting powder / protective

COD-LIVER OIL *(Oleum morrhuae):* alterative / nutrient

COFFEE *(Coffea):* coronary dilator / diuretic / stimulant

COLICROOT *(Dioscorea):* antispasmodic

COLTSFOOT *(Tussilago):* anticatarrhal / antitussive / demulcent / expectorant

COLUMBO *(Jateorhiza columba):* stomachic / tonic

COMFREY ROOT *(Symphytum):* anticatarrhal / demulcent / dermetic / vulnerary

COMMON ALDER *(Alnus):* alterative / astringent / tonic

COMMON MILKWEED *(Asclepias cornuti):* cardiant / diuretic / vermifuge

CONEFLOWER *(Echinacea):* alterative / antibiotic / antiseptic / tonic

COPAIBA *(Copaifera; also called oil of Brazil):* antiseptic

CORALROOT *(Corallorhiza):* diaphoretic / tonic

CORIANDER SEEDS *(Coriandrum):* cardiant / carminative / nervine / stimulant / stomachic

CORN SILK *(Zea mays):* anodyne / diuretic / sedative

CORN SMUT *(Ustilago maydis):* emmenagogue / oxytocic / stimulant

COTTON OIL *(Oleum tigli):* proteolytic enzymes / pustulant

COTTON-ROOT BARK *(Gossypium):* abortifacient / ecbolic / emmenagogue / pustulant / vesicant

COUCH GRASS *(Triticum repens; also called dog grass):* aperient / cathartic / demulcent / diuretic / purgative

CRANESBILL *(Geranium):* astringent / hemostatic

CREOSOTE *(Creosotum):* anodyne / antiseptic / deodorant / expectorant

CUBEBS *(Piper cubeba):* astringent / carminative / expectorant / stomachic

CUCUMBER *(Cucumis):* diuretic / anthelmintic

CULVER'S ROOT *(Leptandra verginica; also called Veronica):* cardiant / cathartic / cholagogue

CUMIN SEEDS AND FRUIT *(Cuminum):* antispasmodic / carminative

DAISY *(Chrysanthemum leucanthemum):* anhydrotic / antispasmodic / aromatic / diuretic / stomachic / tonic

DANDELION ROOT *(Taraxacum):* alterative / antisyphilitic / aperient / choleretic / diuretic / stomachic / tonic

*DEADLY NIGHTSHADE: see *Belladonna*

DIASTASE *(Diastasum):* amylolytic

DOG GRASS: see *couch grass*

DOGWOOD *(Cornus):* alterative / antiperiodic

DRAGONROOT: see *jack-in-the-pulpit*

DULSE *(Rhodymenia):* antirheumatic

DWARF ELDER *(Halymenia palymatus):* alterative / diaphoretic / digestant / diuretic / stimulant / stomachic / tonic

*EAGLE VINE BARK *(Conolobus condurango):* alterative / diuretic / stomachic

ELDER ROOT *(Sambucus):* emulsifier / stimulant

ELECAMPANE ROOT *(Inula):* alterative / antiseptic / astringent / diaphoretic / diuretic / expectorant / stomachic / tonic

ELM BARK *(Ulmus):* demulcent / emollient

*ERGOT *(Secale cornutum):* emmenagogue / hemostatic / oxytocic

EUCALYPTUS *(Eucalyptus;* also called *blue gum):* antiperiodic / antiseptic / deodorant / vehicle / vesicant

EVENING PRIMROSE *(Oenothera):* stimulant

EYEBRIGHT *(Euphrasia):* astringent / vasoconstrictor

FEMALE FERN *(Polypodium vulgare):* anthelmintic / purgative

FENNEL *(Foeniculum):* carminative / corrigent / flavoring agent / stimulant

FEVERFEW *(Chrysanthemum parthenium):* carminative / emmenagogue / stimulant / tonic / vermifuge

FIREWEED *(Erechtites):* carminative / diuretic / expectorant

FISHBERRIES *(Anamita cocculus):* tineacide

FLAXSEED *(Linum):* antiphlogistic / demulcent / discutient / emollient / laxative / lenitive / vehicle

*FLY AGARIC *(Amanita muscaria):* cardiac depressant / depressant / diaphoretic / miotic / sialagogue / vasodilator

*FOXGLOVE *(Digitalis):* cardiant

FRAGRANT SUMAC *(Rhus aromatica):* astringent

FRINGE TREE *(Chionanthus):* cholagogue

GARDEN RUE *(Ruta):* anthelmintic / antiarteriosclerotic / antispasmodic / carminative / stimulant

GARDEN SAGE *(Salvia):* carminative / condiment / diuretic / stimulant / tonic

GARLIC *(Allium):* antiphlogistic / depressant / digestant / expectorant / revulsant / rubefacient / stimulant / stomachic / vasodilator

GENTIAN ROOT *(Gentiana):* digestant / stomachic / tonic / vehicle

GERMAN CHAMOMILE: see *chamomile*

GINGER *(Zingiber):* anticatarrhal / antispasmodic / carminative / condiment / diaphoretic / rubefacient / stimulant

GINSENG *(Panax):* digestant / stimulant / stomachic

GOLDENSEAL *(Hydrastis):* alterative / astringent / tonic

GRAVELROOT *(Eupatorium purpureum):* diuretic / tonic

GRAVELWEED *(Epigaea repens):* antispasmodic / diuretic / tonic

GREEN HELLEBORE *(Veratrum viride):* antispasmodic / depressant / febrifuge

GUAIAC WOOD *(Guaiacum):* antiseptic / diaphoretic (root) / diuretic / expectorant

GUARANA *(Paullinia cupana):* stimulant

GUM ARABIC *(Acacia):* anticatarrhal / demulcent / emulsifier / mucilage / vehicle

GUM PLANT *(Grindelia):* expectorant / stimulant

HEAL-ALL *(Collinsonia canadensis):* dermetic (see *Saint-John's-wort*)

HEMLOCK *(Abies canadensis):* antiseptic / astringent / expectorant / stimulant

*HEMLOCK, POISON: see *poison hemlock*

*HEMP *(Cannabis;* also called *marijuana):* anodyne / diaphoretic / narcotic / nervine

*HENBANE *(Hyoscyamus):* anodyne / antispasmodic / calmative / cycloplegic / hypnotic / mydriatic / narcotic / sedative
(Highly toxic; never take without a physician's prescription)

HOLLYHOCK *(Althaea rosea):* anticatarrhal / diuretic / emollient / emulsifier

HOLY THISTLE *(Carduus benedicta):* diaphoretic / stimulant / tonic

HONEY *(Mel):* demulcent / hemostatic / laxative / nutrient / vehicle

HOPS *(Humulus):* anaphrodisiac / anodyne / digestant / nervine / sedative / tonic

HOREHOUND *(Marrubium):* cathartic / diaphoretic / diuretic / emetic / expectorant / stimulant / stomachic / tonic

HORSE CHESTNUT *(Aesculus hippocastanum):* astringent / vasoconstrictor

HORSEMINT *(Monarda):* anthelmintic / antitussive / carminative / counterirritant / diaphoretic / rubefacient / stimulant

HORSE NETTLE *(Solanum carolinense):* antispasmodic

HORSETAIL: see *shave grass*

HUCKLEBERRY *(Gaylussacia):* aromatic / demulcent / laxative

*INDIAN TOBACCO *(Lobelia;* also called *lobelia):* antiphlogistic / antispasmodic / depressant / discutient / emetic / expectorant / stimulant

*INDIGO WEED *(Baptisia):* alterative / discutient / emetic / emetocathartic / laxative / stimulant / vasodilator

IPECAC *(Cephaelis ipecacuanha):* emetic / expectorant

*IRIS: see *blue flag*

JABORANDI *(Pilocarpus):* diaphoretic / miotic / sialagogue

JACK-IN-THE-PULPIT *(Arisaema;* also called *dragon root):* respiratory vasoconstrictor

JALAPA RESIN *(Exogonium purga):* hydragogue / proteolytic enzyme

JAMAICA DOGWOOD *(Piscidia):* analgesic / narcotic

*JIMSONWEED *(Datura stramonium):* anodyne / antispasmodic / mydriatic / narcotic / sedative
(Highly toxic; never take without a doctor's prescription)

JUNIPER *(Juniperus;* oil also known as *oil of Cade):* antiseptic (tar oil) / diuretic (berries) / parasiticide (tar oil) / stimulant (berries) / stomachic (berries) / vasodilator (berries)

KAVAKAVA *(Piper methysticum):* antiseptic / diuretic / expectorant / tonic

KELP *(Fucus serratus):* alterative / stimulant

KHELLA *(Ammi visnaga):* antispasmodic / cardiant / sedative / vasodilator

KINO *(Pterocarpus):* astringent / germicide

KOLA NUT *(Sterculia;* also called *bissy bissy):* stimulant / vasodilator

KOUSSO *(Brayera):* cathartic / taeniacide / vermifuge

LARD *(Adeps):* emollient / lubricant / vehicle

LARGE FLOWERING SPURGE *(Euphorbia corollata):* antiseptic / astringent / cathartic / emetic

LARKSPUR *(Delphinium):* antispasmodic

LAVENDER *(Lavandula):* antirheumatic / cardiant / carminative / flavoring agent / nervine / perfume / sedative / stimulant

LEAFCUP *(Uredalia):* alterative / discutient / stimulant

LEMON *(Citrus limon):* anticatarrhal / antiscorbutic / carminative / corrigent / diaphoretic / diuretic / expectorant / febrifuge / flavoring agent / nutrient / refrigerant / stimulant / stomachic / vehicle

LEOPARD'S-BANE: see *arnica*

LETTUCE OPIUM *(Lactucarium):* anodyne / sedative

LICORICE ROOT *(Glycyrrhiza glaba typica):* demulcent / digestant / expectorant / laxative / lenitive

LIFEROOT *(Senecio aureus;* also squaw-weed): diuretic / emmenagogue / stimulant / tonic

LILY OF THE VALLEY *(Convollaria):* cardiant / diuretic

LILY ROOT *(Nymphaea odorata):* astringent / demulcent

LINDEN FLOWERS *(Tilia):* febrifuge / nervine

LIVERWORT *(Anemone hepatica):* astringent / choleretic / expectorant

*LOBELIA: see *Indian tobacco*

LUNGWORT *(Sticta pulmonaria):* antirheumatic / antitussive / expectorant

MALE FERN *(Dryopteris filix-mas):* anthelmintic / cardiac depressant
(For use with animals only; female fern is for human use.)

MANACA *(Brunfelsia hopeana):* alterative / antisyphilitic / diuretic

*MANDRAKE ROOT *(Podophyllum):* cholagogue / hydragogue / proteolytic enzyme

MANGO *(Mangifera):* astringent / hemostatic

MANNA *(Fraxinus ornus):* demulcent / expectorant / laxative / nutrient

MARIGOLD *(Calendula):* aromatic / dusting powder (borated marigold) / stimulant / vulnerary

*MARIJUANA: see *hemp*

MARJORAM *(Origanum):* aromatic / dermetic / tonic / vasodilator (Especially good for external use with warm oil as a liniment for bruises, weak capillaries, sprains)

MARSHMALLOW ROOT *(Althaea officinalis):* anticatarrhal / astringent / demulcent / lenitive

MATICO LEAVES *(Piper angustifolium):* astringent / stimulant / tonic

MEADOW ANEMONE *(Pulsatilla;* also called *pasqueflower):* alterative / anodyne / diuretic / emmenagogue / nervine / sedative

MEADOW SAFFRON *(Colchicum):* analgesic / antirheumatic / rubefacient

MENTHOL *(Menthal piperita):* anesthetic / antiseptic / carminative / refrigerant / rubefacient / stimulant

*MISTLETOE *(Viscum):* oxytocic / stimulant

MONKSHOOD: see *aconite*

MOTHERWORT *(Leonurus):* anodyne / antispasmodic / emmenagogue

MOUNTAIN LAUREL *(Kalmia):* alterative / astringent / sedative

MULBERRY *(Morus):* cathartic / febrifuge / vermifuge

MULLEIN *(Verbascum):* anticatarrhal / antitussive / demulcent / diuretic / expectorant / sedative (Do not draw as a tea; boil thoroughly in milk, and then add a demulcent and an aromatic.)

MUSKROOT *(Ferula sumbul):* antispasmodic / carminative / nervine / stimulant

MYRRH *(Commiphora):* antiseptic / astringent / digestant / stimulant / stomachic / vulnerary

MYRTLE: see *bayberry*

NERVEROOT: see *yellow lady's-slipper*

NETTLE *(Urtica):* astringent / diuretic / expectorant (Good for female organs, poison ivy, and poison oak)

NEW JERSEY TEA *(Ceanothus):* alterative / astringent / sedative

NUTGALLS *(Quercus infectorius):* astringent / hemostatic

NUTMEG *(Myristica):* antinauseant / carminative / condiment / depressant / parasiticide

NUX VOMICA: see *Quaker buttons*

OATS *(Avena):* nervine / nutrient / stimulant

OHIO BUCKEYE *(Aesculus glabra):* stimulant

OIL OF TURPENTINE: see *turpentine*

OLIVE OIL *(Oleum olivae):* anticatarrhal (with castor oil) / demulcent / emollient / laxative / nutrient

ONION *(Allium cepa):* antiphlogistic / expectorant / rubefacient / stimulant / tonic (Use for colic in babies by rubbing one-half onion dipped in hot oil on stomach.)

OREGON GRAPEROOT *(Berberis aquifolium):* alterative / choleretic / detergent / digestant / tonic

PALE CATECHU *(Uncaria gambir):* antiseptic / astringent

PANSY *(Viola tricolor):* laxative / tonic

PAPAIN (papaya enzyme): digestant

PAREIRA ROOT *(Chondodendron):* anodyne / antipyretic / diuretic

PARSLEY SEEDS *(Petroselinum):* carminative / diuretic (leaves) / emmenagogue / sedative / stimulant

PASQUEFLOWER: see *meadow anemone*

PASSIONFLOWER *(Passiflora):* antispasmodic / aromatic / hypnotic / nervine / sedative

PEACH TREE LEAVES *(Amygdalus):* astringent / carminative

*PENNYROYAL *(Hedeoma):* antispasmodic / carminative / corrigent / diaphoretic / emmenagogue / febrifuge / insecticide / stimulant

PEPPERMINT *(Mentha piperita):* anodyne / carminative / condiment / digestant / stimulant

PEPSIN: digestant / purgative (Obtained from stomach of sus scrofa domesticus or common hog)

PERUVIAN BARK *(Cinchona;* source of quinine): analgesic / antibiotic / antimalarial / antiperiodic / antirheumatic / oxytocic / stomachic / tonic

PHEASANT'S-EYE *(Adonis):* depressant / vasoconstrictor

PICHI *(Fabiana):* astringent

PILL-BEARING SPURGE *(Euphorbia pilulifera):* antispasmodic / expectorant / sedative

PINE TAR *(Pix liquida):* antiseptic / expectorant / irritant / parasiticide

PIPSISSEWA *(Chimaphila):* alterative / diuretic / tonic

PLEURISY ROOT *(Asclepias tuberosa):* anthelmintic / diaphoretic / stimulant

*POISON HEMLOCK *(Conium):* antispasmodic / hypnotic / sedative
(Extremely toxic; do not take without doctor's prescription)

POISON IVY *(Rhus toxicodendron):* depressant / stimulant

POKEROOT *(Phytolacca):* alterative / emetocathartic / proteolytic enzyme

POMEGRANATE ROOT BARK *(Punica granatum):* anthelmintic / vermifuge

PRICKLY ASH *(Xanthoxylum):* alterative / antispasmodic / carminative /
diaphoretic / sialagogue / tonic

PRIMROSE *(Primula):* calmative / nervine

PRIVET *(Ligustrum):* astringent

PSYLLIUM SEEDS *(Plantago psyllium):* laxative

PUMPKIN SEEDS *(Cucurbita pepo):* diuretic / vermifuge

*QUAKER BUTTONS *(Strychnos nux-vomica):* motor excitant / stomachic /
tonic

QUAKING ASPEN *(Populus):* anodyne / diuretic / febrifuge / tonic

QUASSIA: see *bitterwood*

QUEBRACHO *(Aspidosperma):* cardiac stimulant / respiratory stimulant

*QUEEN'S-ROOT *(Stillingia):* alterative / cathartic / cholagogue

QUININE: see *Peruvian bark*

RADISH *(Raphanus):* stimulant

RED CLOVER *(Trifolium):* alterative / antispasmodic / antitussive / sedative

RED RASPBERRY *(Rubus strigosus):* astringent / tonic
(Recommended for use during pregnancy)

RED SANDALWOOD *(Santalum rubrum):* antinauseant / carminative /
nervine

RHATANY *(Krameria):* astringent / hemostatic

RHEUMATISM ROOT *(Jeffersonia):* alterative / anodyne / antirheumatic

RHUBARB ROOT *(Rheum officinale):* astringent / carminative / cathartic /
laxative / purgative

RIBWORT *(Plantago):* antiseptic / astringent

ROMAN CHAMOMILE: see *chamomile*

ROSEMARY *(Rosmarinus):* antinauseant / carminative

ROSIN: base

SACRED BARK *(Rhamnus purshiana):* cathartic / irritant / laxative /
stimulant / vasodilator

SAFFRON *(Crocus):* diaphoretic / emmenagogue

*SAINT-IGNATIUS'S-BEAN *(Strychnas ignatia):* stimulant / tonic

SAINT-JOHN'S-WORT *(Hypericum):* alterative / astringent / dermetic
(with sweet fern, heal-all, and witch hazel in a Vaseline base) / diuretic /
nervine / sedative / vulnerary

SANTAL OIL *(Oleum santali):* antiseptic / astringent

SANTONICA (from levant wormseed): anthelmintic / diuretic

SARSAPARILLA *(Smilax):* antirheumatic / carminative / tonic

SASSAFRAS *(Sassafras officinale):* alterative / antirheumatic / aromatic /
carminative / demulcent / diaphoretic / diuretic / rubefacient / stimulant /
tonic
(Spring tonic, rejuvenates the blood)

SAW PALMETTO *(Serenoa):* anticatarrhal / diuretic / sedative / tonic

SENEGA ROOT *(Polygala):* expectorant / stimulant

SENNA *(Cassia):* cathartic / laxative

SEVENBARK *(Hydrangea):* diuretic / sedative

SHAVE GRASS *(Equisetum;* also called *horsetail):* antispasmodic / astringent /
diuretic / vasodilator

SHEPHERD'S PURSE *(Capsella):* antihemorrhagic / antiscorbutic / astringent /
demulcent / dermetic / diuretic / stimulant

SHINLEAF *(Pyrola):* astringent

SKULLCAP *(Scutellaria):* antispasmodic / nervine / tonic

SKUNK CABBAGE *(Symplocarpus):* antispasmodic / expectorant

SLIPPERY ELM *(Ulmus fulva):* demulcent / digestant / emollient / lenitive

SMOOTH SUMAC *(Rhus glabra):* antiseptic / astringent

SOLOMON'S SEAL *(Polygonatum convallaria):* astringent / tonic

SOURWOOD *(Oxydendrum):* diuretic

SPEARMINT *(Mentha viridis):* carminative / condiment / diuretic / flavoring
agent / nervine / stimulant

SPERMACETI *(Cetaceum):* demulcent / dusting powder / emollient

SPIKENARD *(Aralia racemosa):* alterative / diaphoretic / expectorant /
stimulant
(Can be used externally for acne)

SPINACH LEAVES *(Spinacia):* antispasmodic / emmenagogue / nervine

SPOONWOOD *(Kalmia):* cathartic / emetocathartic / taeniafuge / vermifuge

SQUAWROOT: see *black cohosh*

SQUAW VINE *(Mitchella):* astringent / diuretic / parturient preparator

SQUAW-WEED: see *liferoot*

SQUILL *(Scilla):* cardiant / diuretic / emetic / expectorant

SQUIRTING CUCUMBER *(Ecballium elaterium):* cathartic / irritant

STAVESACRE *(Delphinum staphisagria):* astringent / parasiticide / sedative

STICKLEWORT *(Agrimonia eufatoria):* see *agrimony*

STINGING NETTLE: see *nettle*

STONEROOT *(Collinsonia):* alterative / astringent / diuretic / tonic

STRAWBERRY LEAVES AND STEMS *(Fragaria):* purgative

STROPHANTHUS SEEDS *(Strophanthus):* cardiac stimulant (tincture) / diuretic

SULFONATED HYDROCARBONS: antiphlogistic / vulnerary

SUNDEW *(Drosera):* expectorant / sedative

SUNFLOWER *(Helianthus):* antispasmodic

SWAMP MILKWEED *(Asclepias incarnata):* digestant / diuretic / stomachic

SWEET FERN *(Comptonia):* dermetic (see *Saint-John's-wort*)

SWEET FLAG *(Acorus calamus):* antiperiodic / carminative / excitant / tonic

SWEET GUM *(Liquidambar):* antiseptic / expectorant / stimulant

SWEET ORANGE PEEL *(Citrus aurantium):* carminative / flavoring agent / stimulant / tonic

*TANSY *(Tanacetum):* anthelmintic / emmenagogue / irritant / narcotic / stimulant / tonic
(Add a demulcent, such as licorice or slippery elm, and then it can be used for hysteria, indigestion, backaches, and so on.)

TEREBINTH OIL: see *turpentine*

TETTERWORT *(Chelidonium):* cholagogue / hydragogue / rubefacient / vesicant

THUJA *(Thuja):* antiseptic / diuretic / emmenagogue / irritant / stimulant

THYME OIL *(Thymol):* anthelmintic / antiseptic / deodorant / disinfectant / (obtained from thymus vulgaris) vermifuge

TIGER LILY *(Lilium):* alterative / tonic

TILIA: see *linden flowers*

TOUCH-ME-NOT *(Impatiens):* astringent / vulnerary

TURKEY CORN *(Corydalis formosa):* alterative / tonic

TURPENTINE, OIL OF *(Oleum terebinthinae;* also called *terebinth oil):* anthelmintic / antiseptic / counterirritant / emmenagogue / expectorant / hemostatic / stimulant / taeniacide / vermifuge

TURTLEHEAD *(Chelone):* cholagogue / stomachic

UNICORN ROOT *(Helonias):* diuretic / tonic

UPLAND CRANBERRY *(Acctostaphylos uva-ursi):* antiseptic / astringent / diuretic / tonic

UVA-URSI: see *upland cranberry*

VALERIAN *(Valeriana):* antispasmodic / nervine
(This is very strong, so mix with a demulcent and an aromatic.)

VASELINE *(petrolatum):* antiseptic / emollient / laxative / protective / vehicle

VERONICA: see *culver's root*

VERVAIN *(Verbena):* alterative / antispasmodic / diaphoretic / febrifuge

VIOLET *(Viola):* alterative / expectorant

VIRGINIA SNAKEROOT *(Aristolochia serpentaria):* diaphoretic / diuretic / expectorant / stimulant

VIRGINIA STONECROP *(Penthorum sedorides):* astringent

WAFER ASH *(Ptelea):* astringent / tonic

WAHOO *(Euonymus):* antiperiodic / digestant / stomachic / tonic

WATERCRESS *(Nasturtium):* antiscorbutic

WATER HEMLOCK *(Oenanthe):* stimulant

WAX *(Cera flava):* vehicle

WHITE AGARIC *(Polyforous officinalis):* anhydrotic / antiperiodic / vasodilator

WHITE COHOSH *(Actaea):* anthelmintic / emmenagogue / nervine

WHITE HELLEBORE *(Veratrum album):* astringent / sedative

WHITE MUSTARD *(Brassica alba):* condiment / counterirritant / emetic / rubefacient / vesicant

WHITE OAK BARK *(Quercus):* astringent

WHITE ROSE *(Rosa):* aromatic / carminative / stimulant

WICKUP *(Epilobium):* astringent

WILD CHERRY BARK *(Prunus virginiana or Prunus serotina):* astringent / expectorant / sedative / tonic

*WILD GERANIUM ROOT *(Geranium):* cardiant

WILD GINGER *(Asarum):* carminative / diaphoretic / emmenagogue

WILD IPECAC *(Euphorbia ipecacuanhae):* cathartic / choleretic / choleric

WILD PLUM: see *blackthorn root*

WILD THYME *(Thymus):* aromatic / emmenagogue

WINTERGREEN *(Gualtheria):* analgesic / antipyretic / antirheumatic / antiseptic / counterirritant / flavoring agent / preservative / rubefacient

WITCH HAZEL *(Hamamelis):* antihemorrhagic / astringent / dermetic (see *Saint-John's-wort*) / styptic

WOOD BETONY *(Stachys betonica):* carminative / emmenagogue / nervine / stimulant / tonic

*WOODBINE *(Ampelopsis):* antiseptic / antispasmodic / diuretic / sedative / stimulant (Use cautiously because it can weaken vision.)

WOOL FAT *(Adeps lanae):* emollient / lubricant / vehicle

WORMSEED *(Chenopodium):* vermifuge

*WORMWOOD *(Artemisia absinthium):* anthelmintic / cardiac stimulant / depressant / digestant / diuretic (in the form of santonica acid) / febrifuge / narcotic / stimulant / stomachic / tonic / vermifuge (Poultice for sprains and bruises: Mix 1 teaspoon wormwood in 1 pint of water; wrap around affected area.)

YARROW *(Achillea):* astringent / diuretic / emmenagogue / hemostatic / sedative / stomachic

YELLOW CLOVER *(Trifolium):* anodyne / antispasmodic / antithrombic / discutient / nervine

YELLOW DOCK *(Rumex crispus):* alterative / dermetic / laxative / tonic

YELLOW LADY'S-SLIPPER *(Cypripedium):* nervine / stimulant

YELLOW PARILLA *(Menispermum):* alterative / emetocathartic / laxative / stomachic / tonic / vasodilator

YERBA MANSA *(Anemiopsis):* astringent / carminative / tonic

YERBA REUMA *(Frankenia):* astringent

YERBA SANTA *(Eriodictyon):* expectorant / hemostatic / stomachic / tonic

# Appendix B:
# A Review of the Chakras

## Root or Sacral Chakra

SANSKRIT NAME: muladhara
SYMBOL: square ☐
COLOR: red orange, vermilion
ENERGY: life promoting; vital energy
FREQUENCY: 523.3 cps
NOTE: high C
SPINAL CONTACT: 4th sacral vertebra
GANGLION OR PLEXUS: pelvic plexus, pelvic nerve
INTERRELATING ORGANS: male: testes
    *nutrients:* nitrogen / carbon / hydrogen / oxygen
    prostate
    *nutrients:* calcium / fluorine / iron / silicon
    female: ovaries
    *nutrients:* calcium / fluorine / iron / silicon
    corpus luteum
    *nutrients:* carbon / hydrogen
ELEMENTS RESONATING TO BASE COLOR: aluminum / antimony / arsenic /
boron / cadmium / calcium / copper / helium / hydrogen / krypton / neon /
selenium / silicon / xenon

## Spleen Chakra

SANSKRIT NAME: svadhisthana or swadhistana
SYMBOL: triangle △
COLOR: pink
ENERGY: reserve; love energy

FREQUENCY: unknown
NOTE: within the C range
SPINAL CONTACT: 1st lumbar vertebra
GANGLION OR PLEXUS: inferior mesenteric ganglion
INTERRELATING ORGANS: spleen

> *depressant:* platinum
> *stimulant:* actinium
> *nutrients:* chlorine / magnesium / potassium / sodium
> liver
> *nutrients:* sodium / chlorine / potassium / magnesium
> pancreas
> *nutrients:* chlorine / magnesium / potassium / sodium

ELEMENTS RESONATING TO BASE COLOR: actinium / gallium / cobalt / radon


## Solar Plexus Chakra

SANSKRIT NAME: manipura
SYMBOL: circle ◯
COLOR: green
ENERGY: life preserving
FREQUENCY: 349.2 cps
NOTE: F
SPINAL CONTACT: 8th thoracic vertebra
GANGLION OR PLEXUS: celiac plexus and celiac ganglion
INTERRELATING ORGANS: adrenal cortex

> *nutrients:* calcium / fluorine / iron / silicon
> adrenal medulla
> *nutrients:* iodine / manganese / phosphorus / sulfur

ELEMENTS RESONATING TO BASE COLOR: barium / chlorine / chromium / fluorine / mercury / nickel / nitrogen / radium / tellurium / thallium / zinc


## Heart Chakra

SANSKRIT NAME: anahata
SYMBOL: cross ✚
COLOR: gold
ENERGY: consciousness
FREQUENCY: 659.3 cps
NOTE: high E
SPINAL CONTACT: 1st thoracic vertebra
GANGLION OR PLEXUS: inferior cervical ganglion

INTERRELATING ORGANS: thymus

*activator:* gold

*nutrients:* calcium / fluorine / iron / silicon

lymphatics

*activator:* palladium

heart

*depressant:* gallium

*energizer:* potassium

ELEMENTS RESONATING TO BASE COLOR: carbon / cerium / gold / iodine / iron / lanthanum / magnesium / molybdenum / palladium / phosphorus / platinum / rhodium / ruthenium / silver / sodium / sulfur / tin / titanium / tungsten / uranium / vanadium


## Throat Chakra

SANSKRIT NAME: vishudda
SYMBOL: crescent ◡
COLOR: blue
ENERGY: expressive; volitional
FREQUENCY: 392 cps
NOTE: G
SPINAL CONTACT: 3d cervical vertebra
GANGLION OR PLEXUS: superior cervical ganglion
INTERRELATING ORGANS: thyroid

*depressant:* lead

*energizer:* arsenic

*nutrients:* chlorine / iodine / magnesium / potassium / sodium

parathyroid

*depressant:* antimony

*stimulant:* bismuth

*nutrients:* chlorine / iodine / magnesium / potassium / sodium

ELEMENTS RESONATING TO BASE COLOR: cesium / indium / oxygen


## Brow Chakra

SANSKRIT NAME: ajna
SYMBOL: six-pointed star ✩
COLOR: indigo
ENERGY: synthesizing
FREQUENCY: 440 cps
NOTE: A
SPINAL CONTACT: 1st cervical vertebra
GANGLION OR PLEXUS: ciliary ganglion
INTERRELATING ORGANS: pituitary

*stimulant:* barium

*nutrients:* manganese / iodine / sulphur / phosphorus

ELEMENTS RESONATING TO BASE COLOR: bismuth / lead / lithium / polonium / potassium / rubidium / strontium

## Crown Chakra

SANSKRIT NAME: sahasrara
SYMBOL: lotus 🪷
COLOR: purple
ENERGY: integration
FREQUENCY: 493 cps
NOTE: B
SPINAL CONTACT: none
GANGLION OR PLEXUS: none
INTERRELATING ORGANS: pineal

*nutrients:* iodine / manganese / phosphorus
*stimulant:* uranium

ELEMENTS RESONATING TO BASE COLOR: bromine / europium / gadolinium / terbium

# ARKANA – TIMELESS WISDOM FOR TODAY

With over 150 titles currently in print, Arkana is the leading name in quality books for mind, body, and spirit. Arkana encompasses the spirituality of both East and West, ancient and new. A vast range of interests is covered, including Mythology, Psychology and Transformation, Health, Science and Mysticism, Women's Spirituality, Zen, Western Traditions, and Astrology.

If you would like a catalogue of Arkana books, please write to:

Sales Dept. — Arkana
Penguin USA
375 Hudson St.
New York, NY 10014

Arkana Marketing Department
Penguin Books Ltd.
27 Wrights Lane
London W8 5TZ